PRAISE FOR
STARSHIP THERAPISE

"Garski and Mastin have redefined wellness! From the irreverent psychology information, to the engaging fanfiction case studies, to the narrative meditations and yoga sequences, *Starship Therapise* changes up the narrative about what self-care can mean. Written for folks whose voices are often silenced for thinking too far outside the box, this book reimagines the box—and it's bigger on the inside."

—KAT HEAGBERG, editor-in-chief of *Yoga International* and coauthor of *Yoga Where You Are*

"Larisa Garski and Justine Mastin have created a radical wellness resource that needed to be in the world! *Starship Therapise* centers geeks, gamers, introverts, and other marginalized folks who have traditionally been left out of wellness spaces. . . . [It] is full of creatively adapted teachings and tools from yoga, mindfulness, and therapy that will empower readers to find their personal agency and make change in their lives through the power of stories.

If you've ever been intimidated to step into a yoga studio or therapist's office, or if you think that wellness is only for skinny rich white ladies, this book was created for you. I can't wait to recommend it to my yoga students. This book is ready when you are—to use stories to unlock the possibilities for self-discovery, acceptance, and growth in your life (on your terms)."

—AMBER KARNES, yoga teacher, trainer, creator of Body Positive Yoga, and cofounder of Accessible Yoga Training School

"Garski and Mastin seamlessly connect fandom and psychology, making caring for yourself—and rewriting the narrative of your life—a magical adventure.... No matter where you are on your healing journey, the *Starship Therapise* crew is there for you. I highly recommend this book for those who've felt left out of the wellness conversation in the past. I am so excited that nerds everywhere now have this resource!"

—JORDAN DENÉ ELLIS, cofounder of the *Sartorial Geek*

*

"Justine and Larisa have created an informational, practical, and engaging resource for all geeks who are interested in a new way of looking at their mental health! *Starship Therapise* guides the reader through topics and terms everyone should know when entering a relationship with a therapist, while introducing tools, tricks, and methods through the lens of pop culture fandom. This book confirms to me that geeky wellness professionals and tools are necessary and here to stay!"

—ROBYN WARREN, MSEd, founder of the wellness community Geek Girl Strong

*

"A fascinating and thought-provoking read."

—TRAVIS LANGLEY, PhD, Henderson State University distinguished professor, psychologist, superherologist, and author of *Batman and Psychology*

*

STARSHIP THERAPISE

STARSHIP THERAPISE

USING THERAPEUTIC FANFICTION TO REWRITE YOUR LIFE

LARISA A. GARSKI, LMFT AND JUSTINE MASTIN, LMFT

ILLUSTRATIONS BY J.SALVADOR RAMOS

FOREWORD BY LAWRENCE RUBIN, PHD

North Atlantic Books
Berkeley, California

Copyright © 2021 by Larisa A. Garski and Justine Mastin. Illustrations copyright © 2021 J.Salvador Ramos. All rights reserved. No portion of this book, except for brief review, may be reproduced, stored in a retrieval system, or transmitted in any form or by any means—electronic, mechanical, photocopying, recording, or otherwise—without the written permission of the publisher. For information contact North Atlantic Books.

Published by
North Atlantic Books
Berkeley, California

Cover design by John Yates
Book design by Happestance Type-O-Rama

CONTENT DISCLAIMER: This book contains material that may be triggering, including references to self-harm, sexual abuse, or trauma.

Printed in Canada

Starship Therapise: Using Therapeutic Fanfiction to Rewrite Your Life is sponsored and published by the Society for the Study of Native Arts and Sciences (dba North Atlantic Books), an educational nonprofit based in Berkeley, California, that collaborates with partners to develop cross-cultural perspectives; nurture holistic views of art, science, the humanities, and healing; and seed personal and global transformation by publishing work on the relationship of body, spirit, and nature.

North Atlantic Books' publications are distributed to the US trade and internationally by Penguin Random House Publishers Services. For further information, visit our website at www.northatlanticbooks.com.

Library of Congress Cataloging-in-Publication Data

Names: Garski, Larisa A., 1986– author. | Mastin, Justine, 1979– author.

Title: Starship therapise : using therapeutic fanfiction to rewrite your life / by Larisa A. Garski and Justine Mastin ; illustrated by J.Salvador Ramos.

Description: Berkeley : North Atlantic Books, 2021. | Includes bibliographical references and index. | Summary: "A self-help guide that explores harnessing the power of fandom to reclaim balance in mental and emotional health"— Provided by publisher.

Identifiers: LCCN 2020036967 (print) | LCCN 2020036968 (ebook) | ISBN 9781623175641 (trade paperback) | ISBN 9781623175658 (ebook)

Subjects: LCSH: Narrative therapy. | Emotions—Therapeutic use. | Mental healing. | Psychotherapy—Case studies.

Classification: LCC RC489.S74 G37 2021 (print) | LCC RC489.S74 (ebook) | DDC 616.89/165—dc23

LC record available at https://lccn.loc.gov/2020036967

LC ebook record available at https://lccn.loc.gov/2020036968

1 2 3 4 5 6 7 8 9 MARQUIS 26 25 24 23 22 21

This book includes recycled material and material from well-managed forests. North Atlantic Books is committed to the protection of our environment. We print on recycled paper whenever possible and partner with printers who strive to use environmentally responsible practices.

We dedicate this book to each of the clients
with whom we have worked over the course
of our careers. Without you, there would be
no *Starship Therapise*. You are its crew,
and it is an honor to serve with you.

CONTENTS

FOREWORD

I write this foreword during a pandemic of epic proportion, one not only wrought by nature but also helped along by those entrusted with her care. It may very well be that we are actualizing the Terminator's prophecy when he matter-of-factly proclaimed, as if simply reading from the pages of history, that "it is in your nature to destroy yourselves." The Four Horsemen of the Apocalypse seem to be galloping at full stride, driving humanity, or perhaps leading it into the abyss. Our nonfictional leaders, who have the power to grab the reins and pull us back from the precipice, have seemingly failed us. So perhaps there is comfort in the knowledge that the alternate universe of fictional characters we have created may very well be the ones to save us.

The average person on the street is not likely contemplating that moment when our sun collapses upon itself, when the animals we have exiled to the fragile margins finally exact their revenge, or when we finally annihilate ourselves. More likely, the average person, if there is such an entity, struggles to maintain a grasp on their sanity while managing the unrelenting demands of day-to-day survival. And it is to that latter group that this book is directed.

When I was asked by Larisa and Justine to write this foreword, they were already known to me from the wonderful blogs on Therapeutic Fanfiction they've written for Psychotherapy.net, where I am the editor, and the chapter they have contributed—"Beyond Cannon: Therapeutic Fan Fiction and the Queer Hero's Journey"—to my book *Using Superheroes and Villains in Counseling and Play Therapy*. They had me at mythology and *Star Trek*, two defining elements of our popular culture that are close to my heart, skin (via tattoos), and writing, both professional and personal.

Rollo May, in *The Cry for Myth*, suggested that when we turn away from mythology, we lose connection to our past and the opportunity to define our present. Were Gene Roddenberry, the prescient creator of *Star Trek*, still alive, he might argue that if we turn away from the then-prophetic plot lines of his creation (and all its subsequent iterations) we close the door to understanding our possible futures. As a child of the 1960s who grew up in both the Marvel and DC universe, and as a psychotherapist and play therapist who has and continues to integrate the stories of popular culture characters into his clinical work, I am not surprised that I found Larisa and Justine and they turned around and found me right back. Though I am new to the concept of fanfiction, I am, in all spheres of my life, a fan of fiction and all its colorful inhabitants, whether they leap from the pages of books, comics, and graphic novels or dance, fight, and travel across digital screens both great and small.

I think what has always been so alluring to me about fanfiction and its close cousin, popular fiction, is that their characters and stories aren't fictional at all. Their existential struggles and dilemmas are ours, as are their defeats, laments, and victories. The characters and characteristics of the fanfiction universe are simply our avatars who are capable by virtue of their fictionality to do those things we mortals cannot—fly, time-travel, shapeshift. But in the hands of creative, playful, and courageous therapists, such as the authors of this book, their clients can do all these things and more.

And therein lies the wonder; for in these chapters, you will read of the plight of everyday characters like you and me, garbed in the personae of fictional heroes, superheroes, and villains who struggle with anxiety, depression, trauma, and relational distress and who are looking for a portal, a holodeck, a transporter through which they can step into a more fulfilling, integrated, and connected self. These chapters are about therapeutic journeys, brought to life through the transformative adventures of popular fictional characters we know, love, admire, envy, and sometimes even detest.

Through our relationship with each of them, we are provided the opportunity to boldly go where we have not gone before. We follow Gabbro from *Outer Wilds*, Deanna Troi from *Star Trek: TNG*, Eliot Waugh from *The Magicians*, Ororo Munroe from *X-Men*, and others as they experience close encounters of a therapeutic kind. And in so doing, we, along with them, learn that from trauma may come growth, from adversity may flourish resilience, and from connection may spring hope and love, not only of the other but also of self.

The timelessness and power of the narratives of these fascinating characters of fiction extend from the savage and inchoate past, to the clashes and conflicts of the present moment being played out in the theaters of racism, gender politics, consumerism, climate change, and global pandemic. This is a book about hope and possibility, brass rings of salvation that we may just be able to grab if we stretch as individuals, cultures, societies, and a global collective. Let's make it so, together.

—LAWRENCE RUBIN, PhD, ABPP,
editor of Psychotherapy.net

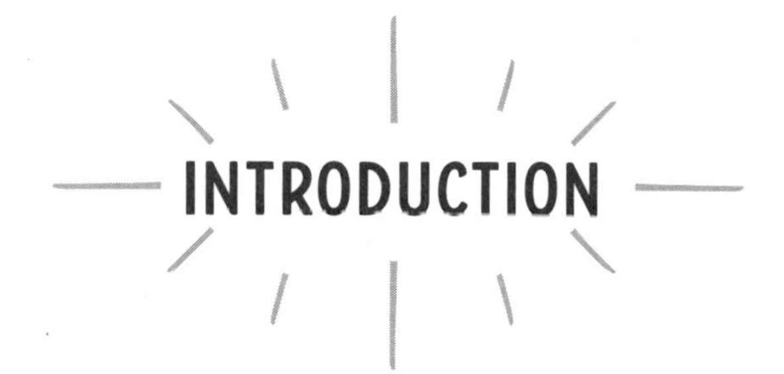

INTRODUCTION

That is the exploration that awaits you: not mapping stars and studying nebula but charting the unknown possibilities of existence.

—Q, IN "ALL GOOD THINGS . . ." *STAR TREK: THE NEXT GENERATION*[i]

This book has been in our minds for a very long time. But it isn't really ours. Or at least we do not conceive of it as belonging to us. No, dear reader.[i] This book belongs to you.

From the beginning, we wanted this book to be a place where you could go to feel both heard and seen. As lifetime nerds and geeks, both of us know the pain of being the social minority among a sea of red shirts. It wasn't that long ago that being outed as a Trekkie or an X-Men comic-book fan meant being mercilessly teased and mocked—or, at best, met with a confused stare and the hesitant "oh . . . that's nice."

Yet even as the Marvel Cinematic Universe makes what was once niche mainstream, the feeling of otherness persists in fandom. The story of the superhero speaks directly to our desire to be both extraordinary and human, to stand out but also to belong. Stories are the fundamental building blocks of human understanding, enabling us to grow, change, and heal.

Though we make use of the extended fanfiction metaphor of us as Starfleet therapists, it might be easiest to understand this book as a self-help guide to the fandom galaxy. For the examples in this book, we chose fandoms that resonate with us as clinicians and that we find useful with our clients. Not all fandoms speak to all fans, and your mileage may vary. As we say to our clients, "Feel free to take what works and leave the rest." You can

---

[i] Here's looking at you, Charlotte Brontë.

also move around this book as you see fit—moving in either synchronous or asynchronous order.

Each chapter includes our personal fanfiction of what it would be like to do therapy with certain fandom characters, because what would Therapeutic Fanfiction be without a little actual fanfic? The fanfic studies at the end of each chapter are examples of ways to enact play and fanfiction using the concepts discussed in each chapter.[ii] As we say on the Starship Therapise, we need to verbalize to normalize. The more we give ourselves permission to embody what we're learning—mind, body, and fandom—the more we will bring it out into the real world.

Throughout this book, we will go over various aspects of your story that you might want to explore and possibly begin to rewrite. You may find it helpful to keep a journal with you so that you can write and revise as you go. For those of you who prefer to ponder Sherlock style, you may choose to imagine yourself writing and/or reflecting inside your mental library or "mind palace." We will look at how society is socially constructed, how fandoms can aid in resilience, and how to go about rewriting your life. Each chapter will conclude with a fandom case study, questions for reflection, and a mindfulness or yoga exercise, all intended to help you integrate the information you're learning. By the end of this book, you will have the power of archetypes to heal and transform your life via the power of Therapeutic Fanfiction!

We sincerely hope that a few or many of the stories herein will resonate with you as you chart your own hero's journey on the Starship Therapise. Whether your headcanon is comprised of dead Russian writers, Jane Austen protagonists, manga warriors, Starfleet officers, or X-wing fighter pilots, the tools of this book will help you connect with your inner strength, create or expand on your own found family, and transform into the hero you seek.

In order to create an even more immersive experience, visit https://starshiptherapise.com/starship-therapise-book/yoga/ and use the password Kirk&Spock! to access videos of the yoga and meditation exercises in this book.

[ii] We have taken some significant liberties in our fanfic, so it isn't strictly canon—we're space therapists.

1

Modern Mythologies of Therapeutic Fanfiction

Elder: Our galaxy has billions of stars. Each of those stars could have many worlds. Every world could be home to a different form of life. And every life is a special story of its own.

Child: Tell me another story about the Shepard.

Elder: It's getting late but okay... one more story.

—MASS EFFECT 3[2]

Have you ever thought to yourself that the story of your life isn't going the way that the writers intended? You aren't alone. Just like any story, sometimes our life stories have a rough chapter (or two): we act out of character, we get betrayed by a trusted friend, or the plot takes a turn for the worse. We can't control everything in life, but we can control the meaning we make from these events—yes, even the "bad" ones. Therapeutic Fanfiction is your opportunity to begin rewriting the story of your life.

Therapeutic Fanfiction owes a lot to narrative therapy and Joseph Campbell's hero's journey, with a nice smattering of Carl Jung for good measure. Confused yet? No worries. We can break it down for you. While you're reading, keep in mind that humans have been telling stories since the beginning of time. Stories are how we've always made sense of our world, but somewhere along the line stories got a bad rap. The pop culture milieu began to get an air of guilty pleasure rather than the status of vital importance that it deserves. Pop culture narratives are our new mythologies. Why should ancient stories be more powerful than the stories we tell today? Just because something is old doesn't make it more correct or more powerful. Whether it's *Gilgamesh* or *Game of Thrones*, if a story resonates with you and helps you understand the world and yourself, then it is worthwhile.

Ship Your Ship

If you're new to the world of fanfiction, just sit right back and you'll hear a tale, a tale of a tiny ship (a relationship that is). Long ago when the Starship Enterprise of *Star Trek* fame was new,[3] fans thought that they saw something more than platonic between Starfleet Captain James T. Kirk and his logical first officer Mr. Spock. They began writing about it and slash fanfiction was born.[4] But that wasn't the first example of fanfiction. Writers since the dawn of time have been re-creating stories to make them "better." Consider how many versions of the *Odyssey* there are: *Ulysses*; *O Brother, Where Art Thou*; and *Cold Mountain*, just to name a few. Aren't they all truly fanfiction adaptations of the same story? And if we have the power to rewrite any story, couldn't we use the power of fandom to rewrite our own story? Fans use fanfic skills to fix stories that the writers got wrong, and we can do the same for our own lives. Fans are experts of subtext and reimagining what could be, so using fanfiction—placing ourselves in stories and examining the stories we inhabit—is life-changing.[5] Yes, fandom saves lives and changes the world.

Great Minds and Paradigms

Before we go any further, it is important to acknowledge that the concepts of race, ethnicity, class, and gender have had enormous historical impact on who got to be "great thinkers." This does not diminish the accomplishments of the thinkers listed later; however, their voices exist in historical canon while other voices are either a footnote or simply nonexistent.[6] Chapter 2 will explore in detail the systemic issues of race, ethnicity, class, and gender as well as the ways these largely invented concepts intersect to create what individuals experience as their own privilege or oppression. It is possible to be privileged in one system while oppressed when in a different system.

Carl Jung was an old Swiss dude who split with Sigmund Freud, an Austrian Jew[7]—a lover's quarrel no doubt[iii]—and came up with many useful psychoanalytic concepts, such as archetypes, the introvert and extrovert spectrum,[iv] and the collective unconscious.[8] Sure, at one point both were younger European dudes, but the point here is that Carl and Sigmund benefited a lot from white male privilege that enabled both to rise from their lower to middle-class status and ascend into the halls of the bourgeoise elite. Race, ethnicity, and gender are related yet different concepts. Race refers to both the physical appearance of said group as well as its social class relative to other groups, whereas ethnicity comprises culture, language, and traditional social practices of a group of people.[9] We are influenced by the gender we are assigned based on our genitalia at birth and the gender we present to the world. Those who are assigned female at birth and/or present as women have continually been marginalized and taken less seriously. All these concepts are invented or socially constructed (more on that in chapter 2).[10] The piece to keep in mind here is the way that race, ethnicity, and gender can interact to give certain groups privileged access to education, money, and success. Jung had some great ideas. And it seems possible if not downright probable that he "borrowed" some other great ideas from his young female trainees.[11] Part of the reason Jung had more acclaim in his life and beyond is that his race, ethnicity, and gender matched what was socially prized at the time. It's important to recognize privilege: the folks who wrote the books fell into the same categories as the ones seen as making the history. But the history-makers aren't the only folks who had great ideas; they're just the ones who were acclaimed and remembered.

[iii] Our personal fanfic.

[iv] Myers-Briggs is based almost entirely on Jung's research (Briggs & Myers, 1977).

Some in marginalized historical positions made it into the canon. During his short but brilliant career as a psychiatrist, philosopher, and writer, Frantz Fanon studied the ravages of colonial brutality on the minds and bodies of the colonized. In such works as *Black Skin, White Masks*[12] and *The Wretched of the Earth*,[13] Fanon, of French West Indian descent, criticized Freud and his fellow psychoanalysts for largely ignoring the African experience and diaspora as well as the atrocities of colonialism. As we continue to explore the collectivist approach of both Jung and Campbell, Fanon reminds us that just as important is the focus on cultural or intercollective differences. The more a person is empowered to engage with the cultures of both birth and choice, the more that person can partake in the shared communal experience of humanity.

The concept that concerns us most here is Jung's theory of archetypes: the idea that all of our character tropes exist in an ancient or primeval form within our collective unconscious to which we all have access.[14] It's kind of like the hive mind but without all that creepy Borg business.[v]

Those of you who are gamers may be thinking, *Wait, aren't archetypes the things that animate objects of power and altered objects?* Right you are! And, yes, we really enjoyed the 2019 video game *Control*, too. While we can neither confirm nor deny the whereabouts of the oldest house, we can assure you that *Control* got most things right in terms of Jungian mythology. Jung believed in the power of the unconscious to shape human perception and dabbled in paranormal practices throughout his life. Was he also a medium? Well, maybe! But you'll have to wait for this book's expansion pack to find out.

Enter Joseph Campbell, the famed mythologist—he was also an old white dude of Irish Catholic descent (notice a pattern?)—who is credited with discovering that all cultures tell the tale of the one myth, or monomyth, which is to say the journey of the hero.[15] The hero's journey charts the growth and development of the young hero from the call to adventure through training via guides and helpers into the very abyss of life itself. Usually, the hero reemerges from the abyss with a special skill or boon that can be brought back to the community, making life not only better from the hero but also for society.[16]

[v] The Borg is an alien race from the *Star Trek* series (Pillar & Bole, 1990, June 18). Borgs really like to do stuff together. You're never alone when you're friends with a Borg.

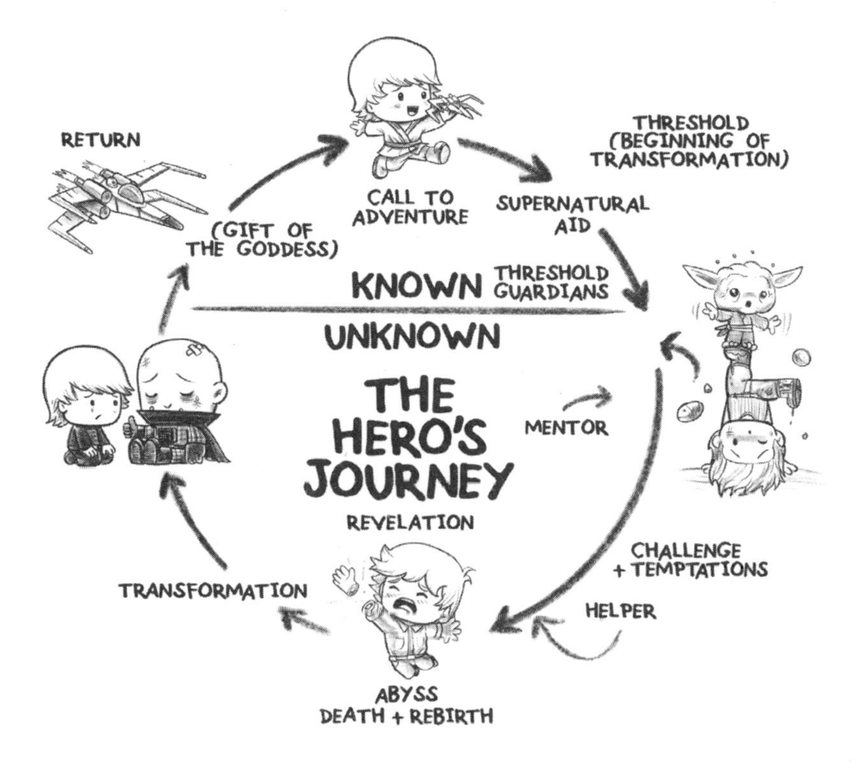

In our modern world, heroes don't just turn up in storybooks anymore.[vi] We've traded campfire tales for movies, manga, and multiplayer games. Although the form of our heroic stories has changed, their function remains the same. Look no further than Commander Shepard of the *Mass Effect* series for proof that the hero's journey is alive and well.[17] The video game trilogy follows the Shepard across countless battles and alien worlds to save all life by bringing balance to chaos. Through the Commander Shepard avatar, gamers join the ranks of adolescent warriors of old who had to pass tests or trials to ascend to adulthood. Joseph Campbell lamented near the end of his life that myths were dying out.[18] But we'd argue the power of myth is alive and well; it just lives in different places now.

[vi] But *The Kingkiller Chronicle* series gives you a great feel for just what those old myths and stories will be like—minus the probability that we may never get an ending for the series (Rothfuss, 2007, 2011).

Next up are some more white dudes: Michael White (an Australian) and David Epston (a New Zealander), the creators of narrative therapy.[19] Did their ancestors originate from either country? No, because colonialism, the practice of going into a region and supplanting the existing population. Are we saying that White and Epston are colonizers? No. We are, however, calling attention to the fact that their very existence in their respective southern hemispherean regions is due to the atrocities of colonialism. Life—it's uncomfortable. Narrative therapy introduced the idea that the person is not the problem, but rather "the problem becomes [or is] the problem."[20] By separating out the person or hero from the problem or quest, narrative therapy inspired generations of clients and clinicians to reauthor the stories that no longer served them[21] and craft new stories that empowered them.[22]

In a way, narrative therapy invited folks to be fanfiction authors—although neither White nor Epston ever described it this way. By looking at your own life as a story, you're able to become the fanfiction writer. So grab your red editor's pen, and begin to mark up all the spots that aren't going according to your headcanon.[vii] Whether it covers events from the past, present, or future, Therapeutic Fanfiction can help you make sense of the world and your place in it.

Fandom Attachment

Perhaps you, like us, have started to feel that this chapter is getting a bit . . . dry? Traditional? Academic? Although Therapeutic Fanfiction certainly does comprise all of the above topics, we're still missing one crucial component: play. But wait, isn't play just for kids? Nay, we say! Play is for all humans. Unfortunately, in our society putting away "childish" things at a certain age to grow up and, well, get boring has been normalized. But what many of you already know is that human beings long for whimsy and look for ways to continue to play. Whether through video-gaming, crafting, or moving the

---

[vii] *Headcanon* is a term developed by geeks as a way to reference their own personal interpretation of the subtexts at play within their favorite fandoms. For example, it is accepted headcanon that Dean Winchester of the *Supernatural* fandom is in a committed romantic relationship with his avenging angel, Castiel (Gamble et al., 2005–2020).

body in a joyful way, all such activities stem from the universal human desire to engage creatively with the world. Attaching to or emotionally connecting and engaging with our fandom favorites is a part of our play.[23] It is playful to imagine what might happen next on our favorite TV show and to see ourselves in that world. Cosplay (it's right there in the name), conventions, and crafting fanfiction are playful.[24] Despite what others around you might say, all this is healthy, normal, and, we dare say, needed.

The attachment that we feel with fandom characters is a parasocial relationship, meaning that it's purely one-sided; we love Chewbacca, but he can't love us back.[25] We all experience parasocial relationships—what we call fandom attachments—at some time in our lives.[26] Basically, this is when we feel close and connected to someone whom we don't know, like a celebrity, athlete, or, yes, even a fictional character.[27] Part of the reason that fandom attachments like these are so powerful is the existence of mirror neurons inside our brains. In brief, mirror neurons engage when we are watching another creature do something.[28] They help us to feel empathy for said creature, which are the building blocks of forming a one-sided fandom attachment. Mirror neurons also help to explain how we are able to learn by watching.

Take for example *Supernatural*, the long-running and beloved television series of two demon-hunting brothers, Sam and Dean Winchester, and their angel companion, Castiel, played by one Misha Collins. After spending countless hours watching the show, drafting copious amounts of Destiel fanfic,[viii] and discussing Misha's motivation with your best convention friends,[ix] you might start to feel connected not just to Misha Collins's character, Castiel, but also to the actor himself.

Sadly, Misha doesn't know you. And really, you don't know Misha either, not really. You know his public persona and what you've created within your own headcanon about him. This relationship differs from friendships you form with other people IRL (in real life) and online, which are two-sided:

[viii] Dean + Castiel = Destiel

[ix] Convention friend is a person you meet at a comic convention, such as San Diego Comic Con, NY Comic Con, or Wizard World. When you spend a lot of time waiting in lines, you meet people.

You care about that person, and they care about you in a meaningful way.[29] But just because the relationship is one sided doesn't mean that it isn't powerful. Fandom attachments can help you through all sorts of difficulties. Even if Misha can't personally offer you support when you're going through a hard time, perhaps watching him portray the character Castiel brings you joy and hope. Or perhaps reading his tweets allows you to feel close and cared about. All of that is meaningful and important. In this case, Misha stands for the guide or helper on your hero's journey.

Fandom attachments can also help you connect with other fans who share your attachments; those one-sided relationships lead to lasting two-sided relationships. Fans have both a shared love and shared language for their fandoms of choice, which allows for a shortcut to understanding. So when you run into a fellow member of the Frodo appreciation society, you have an immediate connection with this other human (or hobbit, or elf) that can easily grow into a lasting friendship. We're not saying that's how we, the two authors, became besties, but we're also not *not* saying that.

An important part of the Therapeutic Fanfiction process is separating the actor (or writer) from the character. For example, you'd be hard pressed to find a *Buffy the Vampire Slayer* fan who doesn't associate one Sarah Michelle Gellar with the iconic role.[30] Not only did Sarah Michelle Gellar portray Buffy in seven seasons of television, the Dark Horse comic-book series that followed the ending of the show continued to draw Buffy in Sarah Michelle's likeness.[31] And though Sarah Michelle Gellar portrayed Buffy like no one else could, she is not, in fact, Buffy. She is Sarah Michelle. We can all appreciate both of these women for their contributions to society and culture and also realize that they are not one and the same. If we feel a kinship to Buffy, we might want to call upon her to help us in times of struggle. The character of Buffy is a heroic archetype that we can embody when we need her. Once the character is separated from its creator or portrayer, we can assume that character whenever we need to become the hero we admire.

Now, are we suggesting that you don Buffy's vegan leather jacket, grab a wooden spike, and head out on patrol to save your town? Er, no. We wouldn't actually advise that. What we are advising is that you use the archetypal power of Buffy to *symbolically* go on patrol against the forces that threaten your world.

For example, if your personal Cordelia is giving you grief, pause and take a moment to embody Buffy. Consider what Buffy would say or do when her high school bully is nearby. Breathe, and harness the power of the Slayer—not just her strength, but her softness too—to extend compassion toward Cordelia (she's probably going through a lot right now; hair doesn't get that shiny on its own) while still holding a firm boundary of self-protection and self-advocacy.

Starting Is the Hardest Part

Let's pause for a moment and reflect on what we just went over. You might find it helpful to keep a journal or digital device nearby to take notes and jot down your thoughts. Some folks prefer to simply reflect within their own minds. Whatever works for you is great! To recap, we discussed the history of stories and some of the great (white male) thinkers in the world of stories and our relationships to them, and you got a very brief peek at some Therapeutic Fanfiction skills. If this information feels overwhelming right now, that is completely understandable. See if you can breathe into your feelings and think of a person or character who has been overwhelmed. How can you right now embody the skills that the character used?

Consider for a moment Arya Stark. You know her now as a brave assassin, but when her story began she was a young girl trying to make her way in a world that excluded her. Arya is the youngest daughter in the Stark family, one of nine noble clans or houses that fight over who gets to be king and sit on the iron throne of swords that looks impressive, albeit hella uncomfortable.[32] After being orphaned and separated from her five siblings (Jon Snow, Robb, Sansa, Bran, and Rickon), Arya survives by any means necessary, vowing to get revenge against those who have hurt her, using her trusty sword, Needle, gifted to her by her brother Jon. As you might imagine, Arya struggles with some intense feelings, which she manages by finding supportive others, learning and practicing new skills, and having a mantra (i.e., her kill list—granted, it wasn't the most upbeat one). We'll spend more time with Arya, using the tool of fanfiction to explore ways both Arya and you can use her skills for growth and healing.

Before we move into our first fanfic case study, a little background is in order on our personae that you will meet in our fanfic. We have been hosting a podcast since 2018 wherein we embody some of our heroes, Captain James T. Kirk (Mastin) and Mr. Spock (Garski). In this book's case studies, we embody these personae and work with our fanfic clients as traveling Starfleet officers and marriage and family therapists.[x] Using the power of the Vulcan mind meld, we speak with one united therapeutic voice.

FANFIC CASE STUDY:
Game of Thrones, Transforming the Narrative from Needlepoint to Needle

While we enjoy our roles as captain and first officer of the crew of the Starship Therapise, we made the decision to take a sabbatical of sorts, returning to the roles that first brought us to Starfleet: marriage and family therapists. We decided to travel to different worlds, with the hope of making new friends and helping people along the way. Our first post brought us to a land of fire and ice. We took on the rather unwieldy post of counseling the survivors of a dragon attack on King's Landing, Westeros. Our own safety assured, we hung out the open sign on our therapy tent with all the trappings, including a well-ventilated small fireplace to warm our chilled clients, and began to work with those who sought counsel.

One evening, just as we are about to close up, two hooded figures appear. The first figure pushes back their hood to reveal porcelain features and fire-red hair. She introduces herself as Sansa Stark. Sansa then

[x] We know it sounds weird. But it's play; it doesn't always have to make sense. And we think you'll like it.

turns to her much shorter companion and requests that they remove their own hood. The small figure, Sansa says, is her younger sister, Arya.

Though we have only been in King's Landing a short time, the Starks' reputation precedes them. However, thanks to our impeccable training at the Starfleet Academy, we know that we have enough emotional distance to treat the sisters Stark. We invite them both to sit. Sansa declines, stating, "I only came to make sure that she walked inside." The elder Stark then turns to her sister and says, "I'm leaving guards outside, so don't try to sneak away or hurt anyone."

We exchange glances with each other, but Arya smiles. "They hardly seem a threat, Sansa. I can sit and talk without eviscerating people." With that, Sansa nods to us and leaves. We invite Arya to sit, and she does, kicking her boots up on our table and beginning to carve an apple with a Valyrian steel blade. Although we typically don't allow weapons in the therapy room, we are aware of the cultural differences between ourselves and those in Westeros and make the necessary accommodations. We ask what brings her in today, and she motions to where her sister exited our tent.

"Yes," we say, "clearly Sansa is concerned about you. Can you say a bit about why that might be?"

"Sansa has always been dramatic. Those stupid romances she always read made her think the world was all ladies at court and chivalrous intrigue. She needs to be here more than me," Arya begins and between bites of apple continues to tell a few anecdotes from their childhood, including a traumatic incident involving a family pet and Sansa's betrothed.

"That sounds like a very difficult situation for the two of you."

"It was just the beginning, really." Arya goes on to describe the death of her father and her flight from home, her long wandering in the wild with the help of a man called the Hound, and her time studying with a group called the "faceless men." There is a lot to unpack here.

Before engaging Arya in any questioning, we take the opportunity to remark on her resiliency, noting that not every young person could have made their way in the world the way she has. She nods.

"Yes. Many of the people I knew didn't make it. There was something that my dancing teacher said—" She sees our quizzical expressions. "Water dancing—it's a type of fighting." We nod for her to continue. "He said, 'There is only one god, and his name is Death. And there is only one thing we say to Death: "not today."' It stuck with me. I think that's what kept me going—that and my list of those I sought revenge against." Not ready to tackle the revenge list, we instead remark on Arya's resilience and tell her a bit about a concept called posttraumatic growth, or the idea that the pain we endure can allow us to grow in strength and virtue rather than withering in despondency (more on that in chapter 4).

"That sounds like Sansa. She's been through things I can't even imagine, and she's stronger. I mean, I guess all of us Starks have gotten stronger—except Bran. Bran's just gotten weirder." She tosses the core of her apple in the fire and stares into the flames for a long moment.

"That's what is so incredible," we say, pulling her attention back from the fire. "You've all been through so much, and you've managed to find community supports and strengths along the way. You even found a way back to each other. Though separated by great distance and struggle, your emotional connection to one another endured. You said that your brother Jon gave you that sword. In a way, part of him was fighting with you all this time." She smiles down at her thin sword that looks so out-of-place from the rest of her warrior trappings.

"I was so different then, when Jon gave me Needle. Everyone thought of me as this little Lady, like Sansa was. She was perfect at it, really—her sewing and manners and all that. All I wanted to do was fight—to be seen as a warrior. I don't know what made me different from her. Why couldn't I just be happy with the way things were?"

"We don't always fit into the story where we're written," we begin. "Sometimes we have to change the story."

Arya brightens. "I changed my story."

"That's undeniable," we respond.

"Would you like to hear more?" We both nod encouragingly. Arya returns the nod, leans back in her chair, and begins to tell us another tale.

FANFIC CASE STUDY QUESTIONS:
Sharpen Your Needle

At the end of the case study, we invite you to complete the following questions:

* What is the story that Arya feels no longer serves her and that she seeks to change at the beginning of her journey?
* What are some stories or ideas in your own life that no longer serve you? For example, perhaps you, like Arya, have felt constrained by rigid and binary gender roles.
* What are some new ways that you see yourself that does not fit into this old narrative?
* Do you see yourself as the hero of your own story, or do you feel like a bit player, a guest star, or a supporting role?

YOGA:
Water Dancing Lessons with Arya

Arya's lessons on the Braavosi art of water dancing armed her with the skills she needed before making her way through a cruel Westeros. Whereas Arya's small stature might have been a hindrance, armed with this style of quick and graceful motion, she became a threat. This yoga practice is intended to set you up with those same skills as you go out into the sometimes-treacherous world, allowing you to feel balanced, agile, and confident. The goal of the yoga is for the poses to fit the yogi, not the other way around. Be mindful of how each pose feels in your body and make adjustments as needed for your comfort.

"There is only one god, and his name is Death. And there is only one thing we say to Death: 'not today.'"

1. You are the sword: Begin standing, or seated in a chair, with feet a comfortable distance apart, with hands at your sides.

A. Pause here for a moment, noticing the feel of your feet connected with the earth, your shoulders broad and confident.

B. Imagine that you have a sword in your hand, but that even if you didn't it wouldn't matter. You *are* the sword. With every inhale think *I am,* and with every exhale think *the sword.* Continue this for three to five breaths.

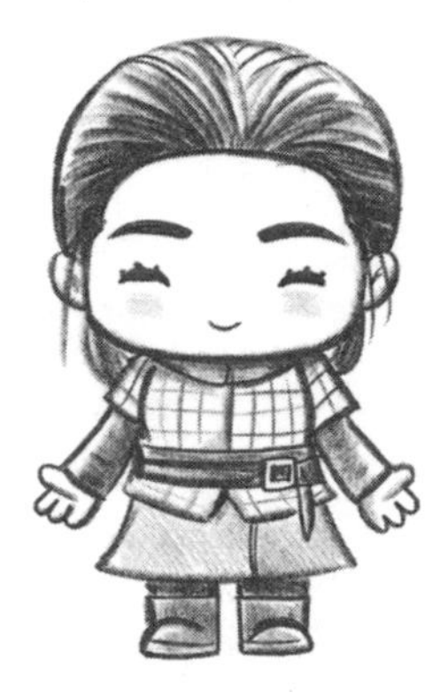

2. Fighting Stance: Take a wide stance with your feet.

A. Turn both feet outward, then turn both feet inward. Finally, turn the right foot outward, and leave left foot turned inward. Bend your right knee. Be mindful to keep your knee above or behind your ankle. Water dancers must protect their valuable knees. Bring your arms out to shoulder height and grasp your imaginary sword.

B. Pause here for a moment, and feel your feet grounded to the floor and your head lifted toward the ceiling. You are both solid and quick-footed.

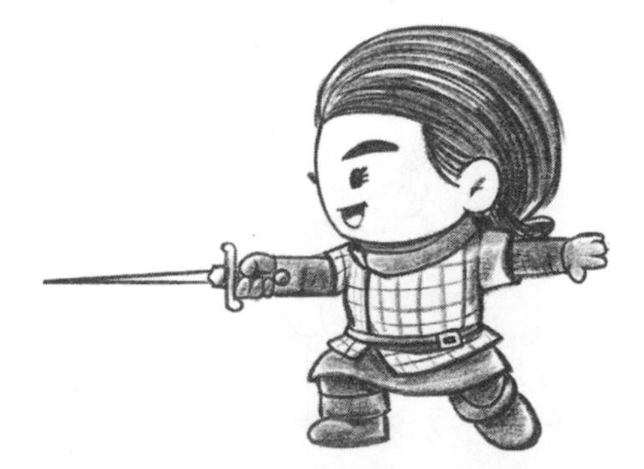

3. Forward Thrust: Thrust your right arm with your "sword" forward toward your imaginary opponent while keeping your feet flat on the floor. You are both grounded and agile.
4. Downward Thrust: Your forward thrust does not collide with your opponent, so you try again by sweeping your right arm down as your left arm reaches high.

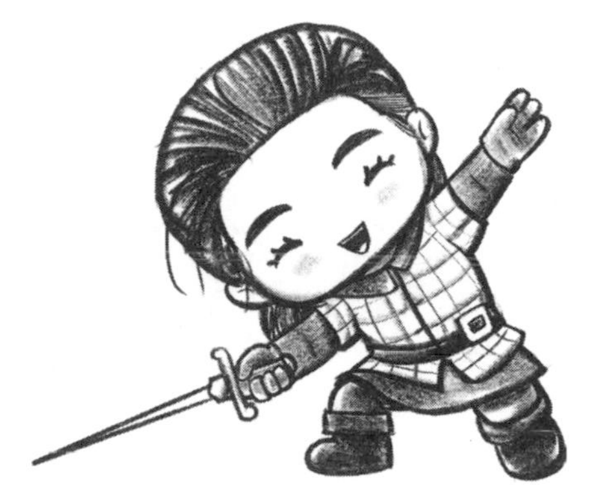

5. Upward Thrust: Once more, show your strength by sweeping your right arm all the way up to the sky while your left arm comes down your left leg. You have made your mark on your opponent, who retreats, giving you time to return to your fighting stance.

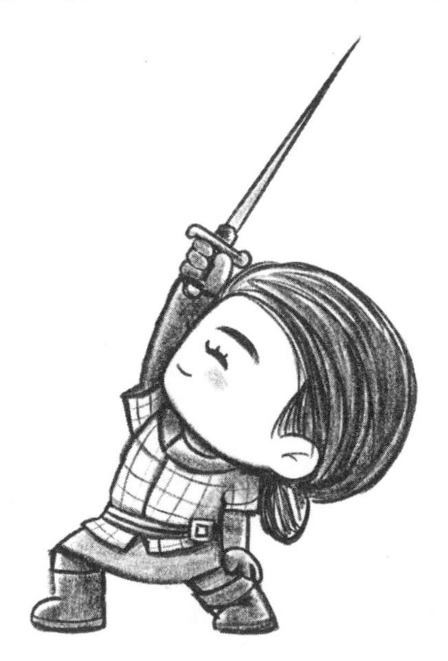

6. Return to the Fight: Straighten your right knee, turning your right foot in and your left foot out and bending your left knee. Jauntily toss your sword from your right hand to your left and begin your water dance on the other side.

   Repeat this sequence as many times as feels authentic to you. We recommend practicing the sequence three times in a row while moving mindfully faster each time. Never move faster than one breath with one movement. Imagine yourself as the graceful water dancer. You are quick and solid, and you are ready to face the god of death and tell him, "Not today."

7. Not Today: Once you have moved through the dance as many times as suits you, heel-and-toe your feet back to your comfortable stance from step one. Return your hands to your sides, or, if it feels best, bring your palms to touch in front of your chest. Repeat your mantra "I am the sword."

The Social Construction of Bodies, Wellness, and Gender

It's all a construct. None of it is real.

—MAEVE, IN "THE WINTER LINE," *WESTWORLD*[33]

One of the foundational concepts of Therapeutic Fanfiction is social constructionism, which is the idea that much of life is socially constructed.[34] [xi] A great fandom example to break this down is HBO's *Westworld*. If you aren't familiar, this show revolves around a constructed "amusement" park where all of the inhabitants are humanoid robots who are assigned genders, races, and roles that can change as the story changes.[35] The folks who construct the park decide what they want the world to be and what the rules, roles, and boundaries of the world look like (more on rules, roles, and boundaries in chapter 8). So the park is programmed, i.e., artificially created to serve a specific set of wants and needs of both the players, or paying human participants, and the park creators. The artificial constructs of Westworld might be easier to spot than the artificial constructs that govern much of our current society, but they are no less created. Very few laws on planet Earth are as inviolate as gravity.

[xi] Your house, for instance, is physically constructed. It's not made of constructs; it's made of wood.

On planet Earth, our social constructs are not created by a team of writers and showrunners.[xii] Instead, they were formed over time. When groups of people live and work together, social constructs or norms develop. They become rules that the society follows, and after a long-enough time, these rules become accepted facts.[36] But here's where things get interesting. Those "facts," as we've seen, aren't facts at all, and they can not only be questioned but rejected. Social constructionism, or as we like to call it, the Westworld Construct, is the way that we see the world, and that can be changed. You can use the Westworld Construct to start to question your own reality.

A classic example of this can be found in *The Matrix* films when Neo[37] is given the option of taking the red pill or the blue pill.[xiii] For some folks, this experience can get pretty trippy, similar to the way Neo feels when he swallows that red pill and realizes that his conscious mind exists in a computer-generated reality while his physical body is floating in a gestation tank. His feeling is both understandable and common: sitting with unpleasant truth is by its very definition uncomfortable. The decision wasn't easy for Neo, though, nor is it for you.

The fact is that change is uncomfortable, and, as a species, we don't like it. There's a term for this in the therapy world: homeostasis.[38] This refers to our tendency to move toward that which feels familiar, even when it isn't serving us and *even* when it's harming us. Change is hard.

The good news here is that, just like Link,[39] you don't have to go it alone. Neo was able to form the greatest relationships of his life and find purpose from seeing things as they really are.[xiv] Using the Westworld Construct can be the first step on a journey of recognizing the story that you're inhabiting so you can start to rewrite it. Here is where fandom can help you. Fans have often been the first to question the status quo and therefore have been on the forefront of social change: the first interracial kiss on TV between Uhura and Kirk being a most famous example.[40]

[xii] We're just going to leave God out of it; Chuck has enough on his plate right now.

[xiii] Sadly, *The Matrix* has been co-opted by some groups to try to keep folks marginalized. For this reason, we like to use this example to reclaim Keanu. He should only be used for good.

[xiv] Plus EDM, so that's cool.

In this chapter, we're going to practice using the Westworld Construct to start questioning some of the social rules, roles, and boundaries that govern our current reality. This might bring up intense feelings. Part of how we change the Westworld Construct is to verbalize our experience to normalize it for others, in turn inviting them to shift their Westworld Construct. The ultimate goal is to raise the collective consciousness of the human species to activate the solar sail.

Maybe you notice some intense feelings and/or memories already rising to the surface. At this point, we invite you to pause and take a few deep breaths. Remember that you can take a book break whenever you need. You can also skip ahead and circle back. This might sound like sacrilege to folks like Spock, who prefer order, but Kirks, who prefer novelty, remind us that the whole point of this chapter is to question rigid rules. Taking a break or moving around to different chapters doesn't mean you can't still live your Spock completionist dreams. It just means that you're charting your own journey much like you would in a video game with an open-world concept, just like in *The Elder Souls: Skyrim, Witcher 3,* and *The Legend of Zelda: Breath of the Wild.*

The Westworld Construct

OK, you think, *that sort of makes sense, but why would I want to question my Westworld Construct?* Great question! There are a bunch of reasons why. The first and perhaps most important reason is that your Westworld Construct might not serve you and might in fact harm you. Nowhere is this found more often than in social constructs around your physical and emotional well-being. There are numerous narratives about what it means to look and "be" healthy.

Pause and consider for a moment what comes to mind when you think of health. Without censoring yourself, what words and concepts flood in when you consider the word *health*? You may want to write down your reflections in either a paper or a virtual journal. Or you may just want to reflect on it in your mind palace. If you're feeling stuck, here are a few questions that can serve as reflection prompts:[41]

- Have you ever placed a value judgment on a type of food? For example, "Carbs are bad."

- Have you ever judged someone's health based just on the size of their body?
- Do you consider the diversity of models in advertising when determining which fitness or wellness-related businesses to support?

If some of what came up for you was related to body size, the types of food you consume, or certain ways that you might choose to move your body, then that makes sense. We, the authors, are Americans, and American society has a very strong Westworld Construct around what it looks like to be fit and healthy based on gender expression. However, this is not unique to American society and is, in fact, a part of all modern societies. What tends to differ are the parameters that govern what is "fit" and "healthy" from culture to culture. In American society, one only needs to open a magazine, turn on the television, or drive past a billboard to know what size and shape the mainstream society prefers. The long and the short of it is that women should take up as little space as possible, men ought to be muscular, and everyone should be hairless from the forehead down.

The media portrays healthy bodies as looking only one way, and even medical professionals can fall into this trap. In America, doctors tend to spend a lot of time talking about two numbers: the number that represents a person's weight and the number that represents their BMI, or body mass index.[42] The Westworld Construct invites us to take a closer look at what each of these numbers actually means and what they have come to symbolize in American discourse. Weight literally measures your mass in relationship to gravity. So if you want to explore your relationship to gravity, weight is a fine place to start. If, however, you want to have peace in your life, perhaps practice some radical acceptance around the idea that Isaac Newton was right, gravity indeed exists, and move on with your life. The BMI was created by a mathematician to be an aggregate to help track average size across populations and was never meant to be used for individual humans. In the same way that we as a society needed some way to know approximately how many children the average family has in it, this math genius wanted to know about what size we are. This was of course based on the common size of European white men. So, it's inherently flawed. But like so many things, it persists because it's easy and it has the heft (excuse the pun) of seeming scientific because it involves math. But it's long past time for this particular Westworld Construct to hit the trails.

Body size is not a predictor nor an indicator of a person's physical health.[43] Let that sit for a moment. If you find that you are experiencing a big feeling, just tune into it. You may want to take a few deep breaths in and out. Now might be a time to pause, reflect, and do some literal or figurative journaling. The truth is that as a species we have a wide range of variability in our sizes and shapes. Not only does this not tell us anything about our health, it also definitely doesn't tell us anything about our morality, value, or attractiveness.

In America, folks are treated differently based on their body size and shape. That brings us to one of the very best examples of fandom that questions the status quo and then sets it on fire and kicks it into the sun: the comic book *Bitch Planet*. Created by Kelly Sue DeConnick and Valentine De Landro, this comic imagines that we are in the not-so-distant future where the patriarchy has won. The world is now run by a team of men, known as the fathers, who make rules, specifically around what is acceptable for those assigned female at birth. In this universe, if a woman (or gender-nonconforming person) breaks enough of these rules, they are sent to an off-world prison outpost, lovingly nicknamed Bitch Planet.[44]

If you haven't read this comic, we cannot recommend it enough. It can be a tough read because the depicted future is just so possible and the comic also tackles some really tough issues, but it's worth the discomfort.

One of our favorite characters in the series is Penny Rolle,[45] because of her incredible ability to question the status quo and be her authentic self despite all rules to the contrary. Penny is a person of color and size who wears her hair natural and has the world's best tattoo, reading Born Big with two elephants. All around her, the advertising suggests that women in this universe should eat little and poop lots (seriously—it's hilarious and tragic at the same time), and she is just living large, eating what she wants, and loving herself. Although these ads might seem over the top, they aren't so much when you think about it. What do ads all around you say? Diet (eat less), detox (poop lots). At one point in the comic, Penny is hooked up to a machine meant to show her innermost desires for how she looks. She looks exactly the same, except she's freely laughing. She wants to be herself and be allowed to be happy. Don't we all, Penny? Thank you for your service.

Now, we recognize that you live in the real world, and not in *Bitch Planet*, thank goodness. But we are under similar amounts of pressure to look and behave a certain way to fall within the Westworld Construct. We invite you to embrace a bit of Penny Rolle and look around yourself and question these messages. Now, let's try out some Therapeutic Fanfiction, and use the Westworld Construct, but as Penny Rolle.

If we emotionally call upon Penny Rolle to help us practice seeing the Westworld Construct, she might want to know some things about these advertisers: "The company who's trying to sell me a weight-loss product, what is their goal? They just want to make money! They don't even really believe in the Westworld Construct that they're selling! Do I want to continue to put money in the pockets of people who are trying to oppress me, or do I want to be happy?"

While we might not all have the quippiness of Penny Rolle, it can help to invoke her brash and beautiful view of life as we move through this. We know that it can be tough to think about all of this, and as we start to ask these questions, not everybody in our lives will be cool with it. In these moments, it's a great time to call upon Penny.

We have now used the tool of the Westworld Construct to question constructs that govern the shape and size of bodies. We've only explored the tip of the iceberg in terms of the social constructs that govern the "rightness" or "wrongness" of our bodies. While we do not intend to explore all of these in this chapter—that could comprise multiple books—we do want to spend some time using the Westworld Construct to explore some of the constructs around both race and gender.

Choose Your Gender, Name Your Race

Race and gender are both invented concepts.[xv] Race, or the idea that the human species is composed of racial subsets, is an invented concept.[46]

[xv] No, that wasn't a question.

Gender, or the idea that an individual's personality and social role are determined by their genitalia, is also an invented concept.[47] We appreciate that these statements might bring up some strong feelings and we're here for that.

Pause and consider for a moment what comes to mind when you think of words such as *race, ethnicity, class,* and *gender.* Without censoring yourself, what are the words and concepts that flood in when you consider these labels? You may want to write down your reflections in either a paper or a virtual journal. Or you may just want to reflect on it in your mind palace. If you're feeling stuck, here are a few reflection prompts:[48]

- Do you worry about your personal safety when you walk alone in a public place?
- How often do you consider the accessibility of the building that you need to enter or the transit that you need to ride?
- How well represented do you feel in the media that you consume? If you feel well represented, how easy was it to find or access this media?

Let's be clear: Once something, like race, is invented and spread through a community, it becomes very real. When we acknowledge race as a created concept, we are not engaging in colorblindness. Colorblindness (the idea that all people ought to ignore racial differences) was and still is taught both explicitly and implicitly in our culture as a way to feel less uncomfortable around issues of race.[49] We are not saying that all people or groups of people are alike. In fact, folks have a very strong attachment to their social, cultural, and racial groups. We are using the Westworld Construct to call attention to the fact that invented concepts like race and gender have as much power as a community gives them. And the human race has given them a lot of power.

Race is one of the main ways that governing systems make decisions about access to resources such as education, healthcare, housing, and capital.[50] Partly because race is an invented construct, over time it has become synonymous with other types of hierarchical roles such as class and ethnicity. The Westworld Construct can help us to understand what race is and is not. At its core, race is about categorizing groups of people in terms of otherness: the main or "normal" group and the "other" group.

The Irish were once considered a race, as were the Jews. Now many of these folks are considered white in America. Nothing changed other than the Westworld Constructs around them. Historically, identifying a race as "other" has been a way to allocate resources amid marginalized groups and keep majority groups in power. Rich or wealthy[xvi] folks get the most resources, and everyone else fights over what is left.

In chapter 1, we mentioned the relationship between class and race and how your place in this hierarchy impacts your relation to power. Now let's talk about how this shows up in the world of fandom. Just like so many other spaces, the fandom sphere has been a tough space for Black, Indigenous, and other people of color (BIPOC).[51] These folks are othered and not explicitly welcomed to join in the conversation. Some cosplayers of color experience a lot of pushback around their portrayals of white characters as being "unrealistic" or poor cosplays. But unfortunately, fandom hasn't caught up with the actual racial makeup of the world, and there just aren't as many characters of color for cosplay. And even if there were, they might not be the characters that resonate for cosplayers. The fandom world is still very much centered around the white male experience. This is starting to shift, but like the rest of society, this movement is slow and requires fans to ask for the diversity they want to see in the world.[52] Remember the backlash after people learned that there was going to be a Black stormtrooper?[53] And that the character of Finn wouldn't just be a throwaway but a major player in the new *Star Wars*? Don't forget the abuse piled on Kelly Marie Tran as the character Rose in the series.[54] Regardless of how you feel about Episode IX of the *Star Wars* franchise, it is undeniable that the endings written for both Rose and Finn were impacted by the racist backlash perpetrated by parts of the *Star Wars* fan base.

Some fans aren't always kind to characters of color nor the actors who play them. We know it's uncomfortable, but it's also important to recognize it so that we can change it.

[xvi] *Rich* refers to folks who amass large sums of money in their lifetime, whereas *wealthy* refers to those who have inherited generational riches to which they may or may not contribute riches gained during their lifetime.

Busy Intersection: Do Not Pass Go

We are ready now for one of the most powerful tools in Therapeutic Fanfiction: intersectionality, or, in other words, the crossing guard. Intersectionality is a concept created by Kimberlé Williams Crenshaw, an African American philosopher and civil rights activist.[55] We like to picture intersectionality as the Zebra crossing guards from Bolivia,[56] but you can use your imaginative world-building skills to imagine this crossing guard however you like. This is your mind palace. So imagine a crossing guard who is here to help you navigate the complicated and intersecting social hierarchies of race, gender, body size, ethnicity, sexuality, class, and ability. Your crossing guard can help you notice the different types of privilege afforded in each of these categories and then help you see the ways they interact to impact the individual with whom you are engaging. Let's start with what we hope is a clear-cut example: Garnet, leader of the Crystal Gems[xvii] from *Steven Universe*.

First, our crossing guard invites us to pause and then identify the systemic labels that could be applied to Garnet. The crossing guard reminds you that *coding* refers to how systems of power label you based only on your physical appearance. Ask yourself, *How does Garnet socially code on planet Earth in the twenty-first century?* At first glance, Garnet physically presents as a large Black woman. So, in twenty-first century America, Garnet has limited social or class mobility due to her race, which means it will be harder for her to amass any amount of wealth or capital. Even if she does, larger society will assume that she is poor because in America wealth is equated with whiteness. She is also more likely to be harassed, victimized, and/or murdered by the police and other white extremist groups. She has access to half the wage of a white man because she codes as a woman, and she will be subjected to increased sexualization. She is also more likely to be exoticized because she culturally codes as other, not to mention that Garnet is a large being, which could be interpreted as being either intimidating or in some ways unworthy. Thus, Garnet is marginalized in multiple ways. If

[xvii] RIP Rose Quartz.

marginalization were a roadway, she has multiple intersecting roadways that could definitely use a crossing guard.

Now let's invite in the Westworld Construct. If you'd like to personify this construct (more on the tool of personification in the next chapter) so it can virtually stand next to your mental crossing guard, go to it! Our personified Westworld Construct usually looks like Maeve, our favorite Westworld park host with an impeccable wit. And what does Maeve say about our intersectional analysis? "Well, you've put on a good show and really tried, but I'm afraid you've missed a few things, darling." For starters, Garnet is not a woman. Garnet is an alien from the Gem home world planet, and she is the fusion of two smaller alien beings, Sapphire and Ruby. To use Earth language, she is gender nonbinary and trans. In terms of race, Maeve reminds us that race is an Earth construct and, as such, does not apply to Garnet at all because she is an alien. However, the way one racially codes is based not on the person but rather on how the person is viewed by the system of power. Reader, you may be wondering, *How can a system view another person?* The Westworld Construct reminds us that the social constructs created by a group can take on a life or power of their own, resulting in a group of humans moving as one collective body or system.[xviii] Maeve and the crossing guard agree that it does still apply to Garnet while she is on Earth. This more in-depth analysis helps us to see that Garnet is afflicted by even more marginalization than we previously thought, since coding as an alien and gender nonbinary trans individual means that Garnet is more likely to be subject to additional screenings (search and seizure) and even deportation. And as a Black trans woman, Garnet is even more likely to be harassed, victimized, and/or murdered by the police and other white extremist groups, as well as intimate partners.

Just like Penny Rolle, Garnet doesn't buy into Earth's Westworld Constructs, so while she does feel the effects of this marginalization, she can recognize that this is due to Westworld Constructs and not her actual inherent worth. Garnet does not define herself the way that systemic power

---

[xviii] See the Borg.

defines her. The Westworld Construct and the crossing guard can help you to better understand the ways that systemic power and privilege impact your life and the lives of others, while inviting you to reject those constructs that do not fit for you.

Questioning the systems that have power over us is part of what fandom does so well, especially the indie video game industry. If you know, you know. And, if you do, then you're probably already thinking about games like *Braid, Life Is Strange,* and *Papo & Yo. Braid* questions not just gender but also sexual politics, using the premise of an avatar who turns back time to erase his ex-girlfriend's memory so she won't remember fights or breakups.[57] And it only gets worse from there. *Life Is Strange* and *Papo & Yo* both question class and race but through very different framing devices: *Life Is Strange* uses a Pacific Northwest boarding school to explore white privilege, sexism, misogyny, and class,[58] while *Papo & Yo* explores race, alcoholism, and intrafamily violence, aka domestic violence, using the fanfiction a young Brazilian boy uses to try to cope with his father's alcoholism.[59]

But this isn't new. Jane Austen began a proud tradition of questioning gendered society that continues to be expanded on today by cartoons like *Steven Universe*[60] and manga like *Ghost in the Shell,*[61] all three of which manage to bring joy and even some whimsy to challenging subject matter. *Steven Universe,* in particular, does a great job of encouraging fans to be curious about gender rules, roles, and norms while maintaining a sense of fun and play that rarely missteps into the realm of minimizing big feelings.[xix]

It wouldn't be right if we didn't include an example from the Westworld Construct's alma mater. Maeve and Dolores, the two heroes of *Westworld,* both take different paths and chart disparate courses, but they share the same desire to be free of the park and the social constructs that bind them. Before we go any further, it's important to understand that both Dolores and Maeve are hosts of the park, i.e., androids, and, like all park robots, their separate actual consciousness—their brains, if you will—are stored in a pearl. A host can be assigned to numerous host bodies of various genders, ethnicities, sizes, classes, and races. A host is not their host; a host is their

---

[xix] If anything, *Steven* leans into those feelings *hard.*

pearl. Maeve and Dolores question their realities and challenge the social constructs that bind them. Dolores has got some great moments. That line about not being the damsel still gives us shivers: "You said people come here to change the story of their lives. I imagined a story where I didn't have to be the damsel." But Maeve is the character who best embodies what can happen for the better when you start to question your reality. Maeve is placed in the small-sized host body of a British Black woman.[xx] After a brief stint as a single mother living on the plains of the Westworld theme park, she is assigned the role of madam at the local saloon. Maeve doesn't stay there long, and as she moves from park to park, skipping across timelines, she challenges constructs left and right related to her class, race, gender, and size. Thus, Maeve becomes an expert at questioning the nature of her reality.

Let's take a moment together and reflect on some of what we've learned. The Westworld Construct is an invitation to question, with a particular focus on questioning those systems, norms, and/or morals that cause you and others pain. The Westworld Construct isn't an attempt to turn our lives upside down but instead to level up our awareness. The more awake we are to the systems around us, the more purposeful we can be in our actions and beliefs.

Self-Care as Activism

You've probably heard about self-care before, perhaps from another therapist, or you've heard the buzz phrase kicking around the internet. Unfortunately, self-care can be a frustrating concept because it's just one more thing that you have to do on top of all the very many things that you already do. Self-care has also been co-opted by capitalism and remarketed to us as something that can be best achieved using money to buy products that will help to elevate us into more privileged echelons of

[xx] If this sounds uncomfortably close to the way one would order a latté, then you're right on track to seeing the horror underneath the "fun" of the parks: a place where you can order a sentient being for kicks just like you'd order a caffeinated beverage. Yeah, it gives us the creepies too.

society.[xxi] But self-care isn't about our purchasing power. At base, it's about the way we talk to ourselves and the daily or boring routines in which we engage. But we'll get to boring self-care momentarily. We've just used the Westworld Construct to question the mainstream message that self-care is best achieved via products. Now let's use it to get to deeper truth.

In the 1960s, there was an amazing African American scholar named Audre Lorde who said the following: "Caring for myself is not self-indulgence, it is self-preservation, and that is an act of political warfare."[62] Lorde was speaking specifically about self-preservation of women of color, who are expected to fit into more Westworld Constructs than most other people. As two women who culturally code as white, it is not our intention to appropriate Lorde's message. We offer it to you, reader, as an invitation to expand your definition of activism. It is true, as we've mentioned, that capitalism doesn't actually care about people's well-being. Systems aren't people. In fact, companies profit off of our insecurities. If tomorrow, all humans woke up and felt pretty OK about themselves, capitalism would implode.[63] So, whether it's to bring down capitalism or just because you want to like yourself, every time you engage in self-care, you engage in an act of political warfare. If that feels a little too much for you, imagine that each self-care activity you engage in is an act of microactivism. We tend to think of activism in terms of the macro: marches, sit-ins, strikes. But equally important activism occurs on the micro level, person to person or person with self. What do we mean?

Imagine for a moment that you were just invited to an event. How do you respond to the invitation? Do you say, "I have to think about it," or say, "Oh, yeah, no, yeah," or make up an excuse why you can't go? Instead, we invite you to pause and actually consider whether you want to or have the energy to attend the event. This may feel like a new approach. If it does, you may want to pause and take a few deep grounding breaths.

We like to think of our energy in terms of spoons. Spoon theory, created by Christine Miserandino, posits that every day we all start off with a certain number of energy spoons.[64] Different tasks take different numbers of spoons, and when we're out of spoons, we're out. So if you have twelve

[xxi] Goop is the most infamous of many examples.

spoons for the day and it takes three spoons to get out of bed, two to shower, two to make breakfast, and three to make a tough phone call, then you are already almost out of spoons with your day barely started. So if the event to which you're invited will take more than two spoons, you're gonna be out. What if you just said, "No thanks, I'm not really into that"?

Did you just experience a big feeling, like you were doing something wrong? Well, that's the feeling when we very first start to question Westworld Constructs and challenge them. The construct says you should say yes and then ghost or pretend you're sick, or some other equally banal excuse. But what if we told you it's kinder to yourself and others to just say no thanks? Such a moment of microactivism can inspire others to question their own Westworld Constructs! Soon enough, your whole friend group creates a new norm wherein it's acceptable for folks to opt out of things, and you might even talk about how many spoons you have or don't have. If spoons don't speak to you, remember that you can fanfic any item to be your spoon. Through your microactivism, you can actually start to change the world (or at least your little corner of it). And when we think about self-care that way, suddenly it's super exciting!

Are you still feeling anxious? If so, that makes sense. According to one Westworld Construct, you should always put other people before yourself, so self-care in itself can feel selfish. To that we say, "Have you ever flown on an airplane?" Trust us, we're going somewhere. When you fly, the nice flight crew always reminds you, in the event of a loss of oxygen, to affix your oxygen mask before helping fellow passengers. That's because you can literally lose consciousness without oxygen. If you first put the oxygen mask on the small child next to you, the child cannot reciprocate. You will lose consciousness, and nobody can help you. We know this is an extreme example, but self-care is very much the oxygen in the airplane of life, and you need to put on your mask and keep putting it on. When other passengers see you doing it, they will realize it's safe for them to do too. You could be saving metaphorical flight passengers wherever you go.

When we don't balance our care for other beings with care for ourselves, we put ourselves and those for whom we care at risk. In the original *Star Wars* universe, Yoda attempts to share this idea with a brash young Luke who is insistent on abandoning his training in favor of saving his friends.[65]

Yoda insists that Luke is not ready and that by rushing to his friends, he will put them in more danger. Secure your own oxygen mask, dude! But Luke doesn't listen and nearly gets everyone killed.[xxii] A construct often modeled for women and minorities teaches that self-care is selfish; sacrificing for the ones you love is important or divine. Using the Westworld Construct, we can explore the ways this absolutely hurts many while maintaining a dangerous status quo. We invite you to take up space in this world because you deserve it.

Boring Self-Care

In the same way that most wellness products have been commodified, so too have self-care products. Self-care has become a buzz phrase to sell all sorts of things. Most often paired with phrases like "you're worth it" or "you deserve it," this messaging implies that you inherently lack worth and must produce or do something in order to have value. Let's challenge that Westworld Construct. You are inherently worthy. There's nothing you need to do or say to earn your worth. If you notice a big feeling come up, take a moment with it. In the same way that we invited you to notice what retailers are trying to sell you, we invite you to question the narratives they are presenting.

Consider Geralt of Rivia, protagonist of *The Witcher* books, video games, and Netflix series. Geralt is a mutant, or monster-human hybrid, who travels the ancient and mystical lands of a roughly European continent solving crimes and saving people from all manner of monsters.[66] The Westworld Construct around rugged heroes like Geralt would have him unshowered, unshaved, and generally unkempt. But Geralt defies this Westworld Construct around masculinity with his love of baths, haircuts, and well-tailored leather pants. Just like the Witcher, you might love a good bath, but you don't necessarily need lavish $20 bath bombs to enjoy it. If those are available to you and they spark joy, then by all means, please indulge. But do so because of the joy it sparks for you, not because you feel you've worked

[xxii] He does get a cool mechanical hand out of the deal, though, so it's not a total loss.

hard enough to deserve this worth. You deserve a joy-sparking bath simply because you are. Geralt doesn't always slay the monster, but he still needs a bath, as does Roach, his faithful steed. Horses matter too. This goes for all of the boring self-care, like toothbrushing and sleeping and eating food. These activities aren't in themselves sexy or flashy; we just need to do them. We are also absolutely, inherently, worth the time and energy it takes to take care of ourselves.

The Power of Mindful Movement

We've questioned a lot of constructs in this chapter. And you'd be forgiven for feeling a bit tired at this point. Questioning reality can do that to a person. Let's shine a light on mindful movement. Notice how we did not use the word *exercise*. Though once a neutral term, *exercise* as both a verb and a noun has come to be associated with body shaping and all of the shame and guilt that goes along with trying to force your body into shapes and poses instead of first exploring *what* movement feels restorative to *your* body.

Throughout history, yoga has been a study in duality: it has been used to invite calm and presence into our physical existence and has also been deployed by those in power to control people.[67] Because we are firm believers in Therapeutic Fanfiction, we get the opportunity to take those things that serve us, like the healing power of yoga, and choose to leave the rest. At its core, yoga is about mindfully moving our bodies and accepting them for where they are in the moment. Yoga invites us to slow down, or speed up, and just be in our bodies. Its focus on breath work, grounding, and compassionate acceptance helps us to feel at peace in a chaotic universe.[xxiii]

We invite you to take some time here and consider the following: what movement speaks to your body? Notice that we aren't asking what movement you grew up learning or what movement you think you should be asking your body to do. If this feels challenging, that's pretty common. Most of us were not raised to notice the movement calling to our body;

[xxiii] Shout out to the *Lovers in Dangerous Spacetime* fans!

instead, we were taught to "just do it" and muscle into postures, activities, and games. If you are feeling stuck, it might help to consider some of your fandom attachments. What types of movements call to the Jedi? Perhaps your answer is yoga or tai chi. Karate or judo may also come to mind. How about the Amazons of Themyscira? Running, archery, and swimming are just some of the ways the Amazons move their body, usually with a focus on purpose and joy rather than dress size. The Vulcans, too, believe in the power of thoughtful physical movement—not to achieve a sculpted Wesley Snipes look but to deepen their personal connection with their physical body.

Self-care isn't just one thing, and it certainly isn't the commodified things that we're sold. It's the things that we find truly resonate for us and help us to feel our most grounded: mind, body, and fandom.

If you're feeling a touch overwhelmed, that makes sense. Remember that you can come back to this chapter at any time to reread and integrate this information as you begin to grow your Therapeutic Fanfiction toolkit. The Westworld Construct is foundational to Therapeutic Fanfiction. It is a veritable Thor's hammer, inviting all who be worthy—and all are inherently worthy—to use it to deconstruct stereotypes. Questioning your reality can be challenging, and it is a practice that you will work on over time; it is not something that happens all at once. So grasp your hammer to remind yourself of your inherent worth and prepare for your next adventure.

FANFIC CASE STUDY:
Steven Universe, Reclaim Your Gem

We take a deep breath and look around our office—ceiling-to-floor windows all around, including the door. While some of you might think, *Holy HIPAA violation, Batman*, rest assured that we are violating neither ethical codes nor privacy laws. No, dear reader, today we find ourselves floating above Beach City in an office crafted by the Crystal Gems themselves—Garnet, Amethyst, and Pearl. But not Steven—at least not today. Today we await the arrival of the three original Crystal Gems for a requested family therapy session. Garnet requested the meeting, explaining, "I don't really know how long we'll need you. Would you be willing to stay for the duration? Beach City is a lovely place to vacation."

Of course, we couldn't agree fast enough. Not only were we excited to explore the environs of Beach City—Kirk being partial to exploring the culinary delights of fry bits and donuts, while Spock was looking forward to beach reading more literature of the dead Russian variety—but we were admittedly curious to meet the Gems themselves, which we sat with before committing to the job.

That brings us current to this morning. We sigh and glance at the crystal gem clock, crafted of rose quartz no less, and wonder if we'll ever get to meet the Gems. "Perhaps we should head to lunch?" We ask aloud to the empty room when suddenly—

"Ugh, Pearl why'd you push me? I was just about to eat it."

"I know that Amethyst. It's why I warped us here early. I'm not going to be stuck in a session with you while your body is digesting all of those disgusting fry bits. Just the thought of human food, of eating, and of the ensuing digestion makes me quiver."

"And not in a good way!" Amethyst chortles as she plops herself down on a plush purple loveseat. "I made this one, see? Yes, perfect just for me."

We make a mental note to circle back to Pearl's distaste for human consumption. As we dotted the final *i* on our mental note, the real Pearl walks up to us. "Greetings, Starship Therapise. I am Pearl of the four Crystal Gems sworn to protect Earth, and you've already met Amethyst.

"Steven won't be joining us today." Pearl's nose quivered. "We hope that's all right."

"Of course," we answer, waving Pearl to sit on an opalescent settee. "But won't Garnet be joining us?"

"Here I am." We turn to greet the leader of the Crystal Gems herself, Garnet.

"Welcome, please sit."

Garnet nods and sits between Amethyst and Pearl on a small red ball.

"Don't you want something more comfortable, Garnet?"

"No," she replies, "this is good for my posture."

We sit, offer the Gems tea, which they all politely decline, and begin session. "What brings you three here today?"

"I dunno," begins Amethyst. "Really, everything's been fine—all except that stupid girl that Steven's dating."

"Amethyst," warns Garnet.

"What?! It's *true*."

"I don't think Connie's the problem here, at all," chimes in Pearl, crossing her arms and turning her head away from Amethyst, almost as if she smells something unpleasant.

"Well, she's not the problem exactly. The problem is . . ." Garnet sighs, looking down at her powerful Crystal Gem hands. "The problem is—"

Pearl gulped. "We're not sure if we want to live on Earth anymore."

Garnet turns to Pearl. "Actually, it's more like I'm not sure that living on Earth is healthy for us anymore—the two of you in particular."

Amethyst tugs at her purple hair. "I'm fine living on Earth. Earth is great. There's donuts and muffins and weird dogs to chase. Plus, I was born here—like Steven. It would be weird to go live on the Gem home world. Pearl just needs to get it together."

Pearl gasps: "I object to this characterization! I am not the problem. If anyone's the problem it's you, bringing all those Earth customs into our home. It's hard enough with Steven, but it makes sense for him because he is half-human. You just want to be human, Amethyst. You have Earther envy!"

After listening to this exchange to get a gist of what's happening, we decide that it's time to interject. "You know, people, or rather Gems, aren't the problem."

All three turn to look at us. Garnet asks, "No?"

We respond, "No, the problem is the problem. And in this case, it sounds like the problem is that the three of you have differing Westworld Constructs." After explaining the concept to the Gems, we continue: "Amethyst, it sounds like you have embraced Earth's Westworld Construct, and, Pearl, it sounds as if you hold fast to the Gem home world's Westworld Construct."

"What about Garnet?!" Amethyst shouts, accusingly.

Pearl turns to stare at Garnet, her opalescent eyes narrowing: "Yeah, what about Garnet?!"

Garnet smiles sadly at her gempatriots. "Finally, you two agree on something."

"I just don't see how we're not the problem," Pearl replies in a shaking voice.

"Yeah, what she says," agrees Amethyst. "All this talk about constructs and different planets. It feels like it all comes back to us not being able to fit in."

We take this opportunity to continue illustrating the power of the Westworld Construct. "It makes sense that the problem feels like it's you. That's what societal messaging does. It convinces us that we are the ones who are wrong, so that we don't look too deeply and discover that we aren't served by the construct."

Garnet looks up from her hands and says, "And sometimes people perpetuate the problem."

We ask, "Can you tell us what you mean by that, Garnet?"

"I'm tired of getting weird stares from Earthers. I'm tired of laughing behind my back when I go for long walks in the mornings here. Did you know that the other day someone actually came up to me and asked if I was a man?"

"How dare they!" Pearl exclaims. "You're a woman and a man."

"I know," Garnet says sadly, her shoulders sagging. "I'd hoped that eventually Earth would be less binary, that humans would grow to become more expansive in their thinking. But I just . . ."

"It sounds like you're starting to lose hope," we offer gently.

Garnet removes her glasses, to look at us with all three of her violet eyes: "I'm worried I already have." She begins to cry.

Amethyst stands up from the sofa and puts her arms around Garnet. "It's why I try to joke about everything," she murmurs. "It makes it feel easier. Like I'm in on the joke."

"What are people saying about you?" Garnet asks through her tears.

"Oh, just the usual: 'Get out of the way, fatty.' Or sometimes they call me a purple people eater because they think they're being funny." At this, Amethyst transforms into a boy wearing a baseball cap. "Or, 'It's so amazing how confident you are.'" Amethyst changes into a coterie of girls, each one pointing or laughing or snickering. "It's hard," she finishes, returning to her original shape. "Sometimes in spite of myself, I feel sad."

Pearl quietly watches her family. She sighs. "It felt easier when Rose was here."

"You always say that," snaps Amethyst.

"*Amethyst*," Garnet chides, wiping her arm across her eyes.

"I say it because when Rose was here, I didn't notice all the hard things about living here. Or I did but it didn't matter?"

"It's not like the Gem home world was perfect, Pearl," Amethyst replies, "There were Westworld Constructs there too. And some of them caused a lot of problems,"

"Can you say more about that, Amethyst?" we ask, leaning forward in our respective chairs.

Amethyst flips her hair and says, "Well, for starters fusion forever isn't done on the Gem home world. It's really more for special occasions, like battles. But Garnet doesn't follow that construct."

"Of course not," interrupts Garnet. "It would make Sapphire and Ruby so unhappy. Garnet is who we are."

"Not to mention the Gem home world's stance on colonization," Pearl adds.

Amethyst quickly interjects, "I'm glad you can see some of what's wrong with the Gem home world. I wish you could see some of what's right with Earth. Like, what's up with your weird food aversion, Pearl?"

"Honestly, Amethyst, I wish you'd just let this go. Food is disgusting and unnecessary for Gems. I just don't like it, and that's my choice."

Amethyst fires back, "Is it your choice, or have you just internalized Earth's Westworld Construct that small bodies are better bodies?" Pearl stares at Amethyst but says nothing.

"Let's pause here for a moment," we say. "Pearl, Amethyst, thank you both for sharing what's going on for you. It can be very difficult to parse out what are constructs of our own minds and what we've internalized. You don't need to know right now. What's important is to start tuning in and noticing. When these thoughts arise, ask yourself, *Is this mine?* If it isn't, would you like to keep it or hand it back?"

Pearl takes a deep breath and says, "You know, I never really thought too much about where my food aversion came from. I think—I mean, I know—that I want to look closer at this. And Amethyst?"

"What?" Amethyst replies.

"I'm sorry for not considering how my criticism of food might be impacting you. I always saw you as the Gem who fit in best on Earth—next to Steven, of course." Pearl reaches out her hand to Amethyst.

Amethyst takes it and squeezes it. "Yeah, and what about Steven? Doesn't he need to start questioning things?"

Garnet interrupts, "Steven gets to make his own choices. That's part of why we fought so hard for Earth: so that the people here could explore and make choices that felt right to them and not be enslaved by the Gems."

"It sounds like you're all feeling more open to being curious about where your motivations come from and you want Steven to understand this as well. The best way that you can model this for him is to verbalize your experience to normalize it for him. You will help to guide him," we explain.

"Verbalize to normalize," says Amethyst.

Pearl smiles. "I like that."

Garnet affixes us with her three-eyed gaze. "You know, I wasn't entirely sure what to expect when I called the two of you. But this . . . has really helped. I think it's the start of the three of us figuring out together ways to battle Westworld Constructs that don't fit for us."

Amethyst nods. "Blast them out of oblivion! Blast the haters!"

"*Amethyst*," warns Garnet.

"Let's just start with recognizing the constructs for now, but later—"

"We blast 'em!" shouts Amethyst, jumping up and down on her sofa, "but metaphorically." She winks at Pearl, who begins to laugh.

"Yeah that sounds about right, Amethyst and Pearl. I think we're going to be all right. Same time next week?" Garnet reaches out her hand to shake ours.

FANFIC CASE STUDY QUESTIONS:

Unearth Your Gems

- In what ways do the Crystal Gems question social norms around bodies and gender?
- In therapy, the Gems are learning how to teach Steven about the Westworld Construct. As his guides, they will help him learn how to question the world around them. Who are the Crystal Gems, that is, friends and fandom guides, in your own life who help you to identify and question stories that no longer serve you?
- Now that you've had more time to sit with the concept of Westworld Constructs, like the Crystal Gems, what societal norms are you starting to question?

MINDFULNESS MEDITATION: Letting Go of What No Longer Serves Us

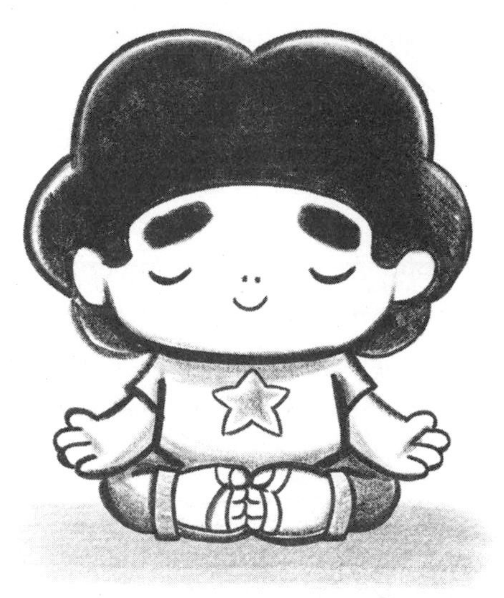

The following meditation starts with the feet. We recognize that all bodies are different and have different abilities. If starting with the feet does not fit for you for any reason, we invite you to start wherever you feel most comfortable.

The purpose of this meditation is to begin to question the messaging you have been given around your body and whether you would like to begin to let go of those beliefs. This meditation is a body scan and is best done while reclining. But it can be done in whatever position is most comfortable for you.

We invite you to soften your gaze as you rest in your comfortable spot. Begin to focus on your breath. There's no need to control your breathing; simply notice what the air feels like as it comes in and goes out. After several breaths, start to bring awareness to your feet, noticing the sensation of your feet. You can move your feet and toes to continue to experience the sensation. Now consider for a moment what you've heard about feet in our culture, what you've been told about your own feet, or how you think of your feet. Are these messages that spark joy for you? Or are these messages that do not reflect your feelings about your feet? Are there some messages that you can let go of? If so, take a deep breath in and exhale out those old messages. Take a moment to thank your feet for all that they do.

Continue this exploration as you move up your body, stopping at your ankles, calves, and knees. Spend as much time in each area as you need; there's no rush. Next, pause on your thighs, an area with much cultural messaging. When it's time to say thank you to your thighs, consider all that they do for you every day, perhaps the best of which is creating a lap for a pet, a computer, or this book to lie upon. Next, move up your body to your pelvis, abdomen, seat, and stomach. These can be very emotionally charged spaces. If you find big emotions arising, that makes sense. If the emotion is tolerable, continue to notice, get curious, and let go of what no longer serves you. If you find that the emotion is overwhelming, pause the meditation, and return your attention to the physical space that surrounds you.

Continue to move up your body to your back and chest. Invite even more release in this area, as our back and shoulders are often the home of much tension. Notice the placement of your shoulders. If they are reaching toward your earlobes, invite them to slowly ease back down. Move up again to your neck and head, paying attention to your ears as well. There's a lot to be grateful for.

Finally bring awareness to your face, a place about which culture has a lot to say. Practice relaxing your jaw and the space between your eyebrows. See what it feels like to relax your tongue away from the top of your mouth. Appreciate all that your face does for you: allowing you to connect with other beings and express your inner thoughts in an outer way without ever uttering a word.

Once you've moved all the way up your body, pause and consider the entirety of your physical form as a complete entity. Allow your feelings of appreciation for yourself to permeate your entire being. Stay here in this place of gratitude for as long as you are able, and remind yourself of this feeling once you move back out into the external world.

Battling Your Gremlins: Struggling with Anxiety and Depression

To admit that you're afraid gives you strength.

—COUNSELOR DEANNA TROI,
***STAR TREK: THE NEXT GENERATION*, "NIGHT TERRORS."[68]**

The time was 1987. The town was your town, our town, really any small middle-American town that also had a teeming red-light district and a father who is also a narrator capable of providing racially tinged and culturally insensitive voice-over.[69] Our story begins in one such red-light district, where a cute and vaguely exotic-looking cage shakes, bearing inside it the cute and furry form of—a Furby? But those won't debut until 1998. The point of view shifts to one beleaguered Billy, a boy who lives in a town brought low by the bust of the 1980s economy. His is a town where adults live in large hard-to-heat McMansions but for some reason do not seem to hold down jobs. Don't ask questions; Christopher Columbus (the writer, not the conquistador) knew what he was doing. In this town, only the preteens and teenagers seem to be employed. Some are bartenders by night and bank tellers by day. Other children chop trees and deliver them to homes in need of Christmas cheer. Billy works at the bank, or is trying to, when his life is overtaken, first by an adorable Mogwai friend, Gizmo (admittedly, he does look nearly identical to a Furby). Gizmo comes with a set of careful instructions:

- Don't shine bright light on Gizmo.
- Don't feed him after midnight.
- Don't get him wet.

If these aren't followed to the letter, he births numerous gremlins, which are creatures who look like Mogwai but with scales instead of fur and more menacing haircuts.[xxiv] As you've probably guessed, Billy does indeed break all three rules, and destructive hijinks ensue.

We are not suggesting that anxiety and its twin depression are actual gremlins (think Furbies on bath salts).[xxv] We are saying that personifying these two most common mental-health diagnoses is a fun and helpful way to both understand their symptoms and start to externalize them.

Externalizing the problem is a tool of narrative therapy[xxvi] that can help you to separate yourself from the struggles that plague you.[70] Just as we would never say "Commander Shepard is a Reaper,"[xxvii] we would also never say, "You are depressed." Rather, in our work with therapy clients, we use externalizing language such as "Commander Shepard struggles with Reapers" and "You are struggling with depression" or "It sounds like anxiety is getting the better of you today."

The difference might feel subtle, but it's important. Part of what neuroscience tells us is just how prompt-dependent our conscious mind can be. Self-talk, or our internal monologue or voice-over, directly determines both what we notice first in our external world and the kinds of memories our

[xxiv] We evoke the story of *Gremlins* because it's such a great metaphor for anxiety. However, the film *Gremlins,* like many films of the eighties, is problematic due to the various "isms" it embodies: sexism, racism, ethnocentrism, and more!

[xxv] Or if you don't know what a Furby is, imagine an Ewok, but kind of reptilian and definitely evil.

[xxvi] Shout out to White and Epston from chapter 1!

[xxvii] Hat tip to the fan interpretation of *Mass Effect 1–3,* compiled in a truly fascinating YouTube video, arguing that Commander Shepard gets turned into a member of the alien machine race, the Reapers, becoming a sleeper agent for the other side.

brain retrieves for us. Think back to chapter 2 and our chat about HBO's *Westworld*. We talked about the ways that *Westworld* masterfully uses the cyborg archetype to teach us basic behavior facts.

For instance, one of the core functions of the brain is pattern matching. So, when you say to yourself, *I'm really anxious today,* your brain immediately seeks to find the other things in your external and internal reality that match this prompt. You might have some familiarity with this concept via the term *confirmation bias.*[71] Human beings believe a concept and then look for evidence to support it. While looking for the evidence, human beings tend not to notice anything to the contrary.

This is where your emotions come in. Your emotions are designed to give you information about your relationship to yourself and to your external reality. Similar to a thermometer, your emotions will give you information about both the type of feeling or feelings evoked and the intensity of the feeling or feelings evoked.[72] Thus, each emotion has a core message and a corresponding call to action. The thermometer tells you it's 30°F, and the call to action is to put on a sweater (or a parka, depending on your unique needs). When you notice sadness, its message might be that you are missing your friend, and the corresponding call to action might be to phone that friend.

Emotions are in fact very good at inviting us to pay attention and notice![xxviii] However, emotions don't tell time very well. Put another way, the Westworld Construct of time as being divided into three slices—the past, present, and future—does not make sense to your feelings. As far as our feelings are concerned, everything exists in an infinite now. And before you go hating on your feelings for their inability to tell time, we offer to you that time is a social construct, but more important, your feelings' conception of time as an infinite now actually maps with Einstein's concept of time.[xxix] So, if your brain is busy highlighting things in your external world that match with anxiety while also calling up memories of anxiety, your emotions will do what they do best: they will respond to these internal and external anxiety-inducing stimuli by flooding your body with anxious feelings.

[xxviii] And, just like Navi, they can be a li'l irritating.

[xxix] Score 1 for the feelings!

Using the tools of externalizing the problem and personifying the problem, you can help yourself identify the anxiety without increasing your felt experience of that anxiety.[73] While Gizmo is connected to the gremlins, he is distinctly separate from them. Similarly, you might be connected to your anxiety, but you are not equivalent to your anxiety. Think of it like a cold: You get a cold, but you do not become a cold.

But if we can find negative thoughts and feelings, we can also do the reverse. We can search our mind and external world for exceptions or times when the problem was not the problem. In this case, times when Gizmo, the adorable Mogwai, did not accidentally birth chaotic gremlins but instead stayed content and warm in his wicker basket.

Let's pause and reflect for a moment. Do you have any mental gremlins in your life? Or perhaps literal gremlins? (We're not here to judge.) Regardless, we invite you to take a moment and reflect on the impact that these negative thoughts or Westworld Constructs have in your life. You may want to write down either in a literal or metaphorical journal some of the metaphorical gremlins that hijack your thoughts and feelings and send you into a negative tailspin. Once you've come up with three to five examples, you may want to consider instances where the opposite happened. Have you experienced a situation that might cause an anxiety gremlin, but then everything went OK? Maybe something you were scared of happening didn't, and you even had a nice time. Write down a few of those examples. We'll circle back to them later.

You may wonder, *How do I keep my adorable Mogwai from turning into horrific gremlins of destruction?* We're glad you asked. Just like Gizmo came with a set of instructions, so do we all have our own self-care plan that keeps us from erupting with pint-sized hellions. For Gizmo, his rules were around not getting wet, no direct sunlight, and no food after midnight. Those are some pretty relatable self-care topics, actually. Unlike Mogwai, we need all of those items for survival (although admittedly we don't need to eat after midnight). Generally speaking, we need to be fed and watered regularly, move our bodies in some way, sleep with some consistency, and engage in creative or meaningful pursuits. Mileage varies from person to person, but generally these are the rules of the Mogwai that is you. Are we always perfect at this? We are absolutely not. And that isn't an invitation to beat ourselves up, just an invitation to pay attention. Just like when Gizmo first got wet, we make mistakes, and our gremlins can get activated. It's important to notice the gremlins early so that we can be mindful of following the other "rules" and keep the little dudes from turning scaly.

Choose Your Anxiety Avatar

Right about now you might be thinking, *But what if I've never watched* Gremlins*? What does my anxiety avatar look like?* Anime, manga, comics, and cartoons provide you with a wealth of options when it comes to crafting a fanfic of your own personal anxiety or distress. Let's start with anime.

"TETSUO?!" "KANEDA!" Does this ring any bells? For those who don't know (or who forgot), Tetsuo and his best bro Kaneda are two of the main characters in the beloved manga *Akira*,[74] famously remade into the anime of the same name.[75] Whether you're into the anime or manga version, you'll recall that Tetsuo becomes an entirely different version of himself following a collision with an Esper, that is, a psychically enhanced human. Following this collision, the once kindhearted Tetsuo becomes increasingly agitated and tense, culminating in a telekinetic rampage. Tetsuo's manifestation of anxiety triggered by the resurgence of latent psychic powers mirrors the anxiety described by folks who are emotionally sensitive humans or folks who just pick up on other people's emotions. As our clients sometimes tell us, "Sometimes I have a hard time figuring out what feelings are mine and what feelings belong to other folks."

If you're an avid gamer, you may have already guessed which recent gaming avatar best personifies anxiety. Did you think of Dark Madeline? Madeline is the mountain-climbing novice in the 2019 game *Celeste* whose literal hero's journey takes her on an adventure to face her darkest fear: her anxious self.[76] Known as Dark Madeline, this anxiety avatar causes Madeline a host of troubles until Madeline tries talking to this fractured part of herself and learns, among other things, that Dark Madeline's panic attacks and catastrophizing talk are misguided attempts to keep real Madeline safe.

Similar to Tetsuo's telepathy-induced anxiety meltdown, Jean Grey of the *Uncanny X-Men* struggles with her own psychic darkness, personified by the Dark Phoenix.[77] There have been many versions of this story,[xxx] but the main point here is that although Dark Phoenix is connected to the real Jean Grey, she is a separate entity. Anxiety often sounds like us—it makes use of our mind just like our own thoughts—but it is not the authentic Self.

It might feel intuitive to you to think about having multiple parts of yourself. For example, right now you might have a part of you that's anxious, a part of you that's excited, and a part that's bored (we're sorry). Our goal is not to help you get rid of your parts, but rather to guide you in befriending them so that the Self can make the best decisions for all parts of you.

Depression Demogorgon: The Depressogorgon

Our clients are less likely to describe their depression[78] in terms of frantic little monsters and more likely to describe it in terms of huge, overwhelming monsters who suck all the air out of the room. The Dementors from *Harry Potter* are a common avatar for this feeling,[79] but in this chapter, we will look at depression through the lens of the Demogorgon from Netflix's *Stranger Things*.[80] It's a big scary monster, and we get to stick with the 1980s aesthetic we've already got going. When the Demogorgon appears, it essentially takes Will Byers hostage. The Demogorgon cuts him off from his friends and family and traps him somewhere very cold and colorless. This isn't that different than how folks describe being "kidnapped" by their depression.

Will is fortunate to have friends and family who recognize he is in danger and try to help him. Even once he returns to the regular world, the effects of the Demogorgon linger. This is the very real impact of depression. It is a monster, but it does not appear without warning,[xxxi] and we are not alone in coping with it. Unlike the *Stranger Things* Demogorgon, our goal is not to slay depression but rather to find ways to keep it in the Upside Down and figure out how to get it to hang out with us and play some D&D when

[xxx] And, yes, we are choosing to ignore both movie adaptations.

[xxxi] Even though sometimes it feels like it comes out of nowhere.

it visits. It will never make for a particularly fun playmate, but it also doesn't need to devour the entire town to get our attention.

Remember that list we encouraged you to write and said we'd circle back to? Externalization and personification are powerful tools that help to separate you from the anxiety, depression, or both that plague you. And, once you've gotten a handle on some unique outcomes—times when an initiating external event happens that usually makes you go all Tetsuo, but instead you don't—then you're ready to rewrite your anxiety and depression narrative.[81] Once you externalize the "problem" and find exceptions, you can begin to think and talk about your feelings in new ways, eventually leading to the creation of a whole new narrative.

Choose Your Depression Avatar

But what if *Stranger Things* isn't your thing? Here's a short breakdown of some other possible depression avatars to start rewriting your own depression narrative. Think of these as a springboard into other ideas. Perhaps Mae from *Night in the Woods* isn't your jam, but Max Payne's[xxxii] revenge depression really speaks to you. We invite you to take what works and leave the rest.

An excellent example of depression in gaming occurs in the beloved indie game *Thomas Was Alone.*[82] Similar to *Night in the Woods*, it is a great game for experienced and new gamers alike. Plus, it's available on every platform. Each character in *Thomas* is a rogue AI represented by a different polygon. Claire is a big blue cube who struggles with depression stemming from her fear that she is "too big." Alone and dejected, she wanders the binary void until she comes across a problem that only her size can solve. Buoyed by this positive experience, Claire embarks on a mission of bravery to help herself and her friends.

This example may feel like a cliché, but it has endured for a reason: Eeyore of the *Winnie the Pooh* books and series of beloved childhood

---

[xxxii] A modern noir video game series that follows the titular Max on a series of violent quests to avenge his murdered family.

cartoons and movies is a common personification of depression. Glum and dejected, Eeyore often sees the worst in any given situation and is the first to advise against fun. Arguably a bit of a downer (OK, maybe a lot of a downer), Eeyore is helped by his many friends who understand that beneath his dismal outlook exists a kindhearted donkey who would risk just about anything—including his tail—for his friends.[83]

Have you played *Night in the Woods* yet?[84] If not, we highly recommend this third-person-point-of-view role-play game. One benefit of this game is that it is easily playable regardless of your gaming experience. Mae, an adorable anthropomorphic cat, returns after a failed stint at college to her hometown of Possum Springs, a once affluent mining town that has fallen on hard times. Despite Mae being profoundly depressed, Mae's parents willfully ignore their daughter's symptoms. Mae's depression takes the form of disaffected lethargy, sporadically falling into bouts of Max Payne–level displays of violence.

Let's take a moment and use Mae as an example of how we can fanfic your depression. Fortunately for Mae, her friends in the game are wonderfully understanding of what she's going through—even her snarky alligator friend, Bea. If you picture your depression as an adorable cat with supportive friends, it's easier to offer some compassion to that part of yourself and to interact with depression in new ways. The Mae part doesn't want to be sad; she doesn't want to hurt anybody else. She's just having a hard time and could use your support. Picturing your depression this way offers you a new way to think about it, a new story to inhabit. When you feel Mae acting up, it's an indication that she needs a bit of attention. What are the things Mae likes? Seeing her friends, playing the bass, and crimes. We can't condone crimes, but what all these things have in common for Mae is that they offer her a sense of meaning. So in order to help your Mae, you might need some time to be artistic, or burn off some sadness in the form of exercise, or, yes, see friends. Suddenly depression is a lot less scary when it's an adorable cat.

Panic at the Disco

Now that we've covered the dynamic duo of anxiety and depression, let's explore one last common mental health issue: social anxiety. We find that this type of anxiety is less of a gremlin, an irritating little creature that won't go away, and more like No-Face from Hayao Miyazaki's *Spirited Away*.[85] No-Face appears on the outside of a boisterous bathhouse, loitering until he's invited inside. He feels so indebted to Sen, who invited him in, that he tries to give her just way too many tokens for bath bombs (it's a bathhouse). In an effort to fit in, No-Face winds up acting contrary to his kind nature, giving out fake gold and eating everything in the bathhouse.

If you deal with social anxiety, you might recognize this feeling. So many folks deal with social anxiety for a variety of reasons, but a reason that isn't often considered harkens back to the Westworld Construct. In Western culture, a value is placed on extroversion over introversion. Thus, extroverted behaviors are the ones that culturally code as "normal" or "correct." The truth is that often what is perceived as being socially awkward is really just a misunderstanding between two different types of folks. The situation is awkward, but neither person is awkward.

Both extroverts and introverts need social time and alone time. The difference is in the method. A classic introvert like Bruce Banner, the Hulk's alter ego, cannot recharge at a club, Tony Stark style.[86] Ironman Tony can dance the night away, reenergizing off the swell of social activity and powering up for late-night sessions working on more solitary pursuits with Jarvis in his lab/home office. But Bruce Banner must end his research early so that he can recharge in his study with a good book before joining Tony later at the club. It might be most helpful to think of introversion and extroversion existing on a spectrum rather than being a black-or-white, one-or-the-other position.

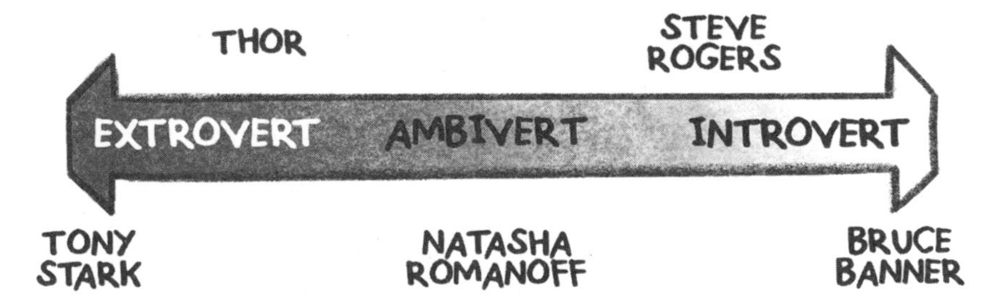

Whether you struggle with gremlins, Demogorgons, No-Faces, or discos, using the tools of externalization and personification can help you figure out the cast of characters you need in your Therapeutic Fanfiction story. Everyone struggles with different problems. But when we can use the power of play to find compassion, suddenly they don't seem so scary. It's like the Boggart in *Harry Potter*.[87] It's a terrifying spider until you put some roller skates on it, and then it's just funny AF.

FANFIC CASE STUDY:
Gremlins (1 and 2), Billy's Malaise

After spending some time in Beach City, we decided we'd had enough of the sun and needed a change in scenery. We set our sights on Manhattan in the early 1990s and rented offices just around the corner from a recently demolished Chinese artifacts shop.[88] After returning from a particularly successful shopping trip for wide-shouldered polyester suits, we had just enough time to prepare for a new clinical intake: Billy Peltzer. Billy is coming in for therapy at the insistence of his fiancée, Kate, who explained on the phone that she is concerned about Billy's state of mind after a recent trauma.

At a quarter past three, Billy appears at our offices looking slightly disheveled with a forced grin and JanSport backpack. After declining tea (we help ourselves), Billy, at our invitation, tells us a bit about what brought him to the city.

"Well," he begins, "I needed to get out of my hometown." We nod for him to go on. "You see, I made some mistakes when I was younger, and I thought moving would put them behind me, but they just keep following me—everywhere I go. Even when I think that I've moved on, I turn around and they're right there behind me—literally. I mean, I love the little fur ball and all, but I can't seem to take care of him the way he needs me to. And he terrifies Kate because she's afraid of what he might spawn."

At this point, we invite Billy to pause. "Who is your friend?"

"Oh, yeah. Maybe Kate didn't tell you on the phone?"

We shake our heads no.

"Well, my friend is named Gizmo, and he's a Mogwai. He's cute and furry and really polite, actually. So when it's just him, everything is great. But the trouble is something always goes wrong, and he eats after midnight, or I accidentally spill water on him or shine a bright light in his face. Ugh! I just feel like I can't do anything right. At first, I thought it was all my hometown but now..." He continues to rehash the events of his Mogwai-turned-gremlins and the battles that occurred both in his hometown and then more recently here in NYC.

"Yes," we respond, "that's a very common complaint. People believe that they can outrun their troubles or move away from them. Unfortunately, they stay with us no matter where we go."

Billy sighs. "Despite all its troubles, I really do love my hometown. I just didn't feel like there was enough opportunity there—even without the whole gremlin drama. I feel like I need to be really successful before I can officially get married to Kate."

"What does it mean to be successful, Billy?" we ask.

"Well, money, I guess. That seems to be what it's all about, right?"

"Money is one way to measure success, but it certainly isn't the *only* way. From what you've told us, it sounds like you've been very successful in other ways. You saved your town from a gremlin attack and then also helped save this city from being overrun as well, which we appreciate on a personal level."

Billy looks down at his hands. "I guess. I just don't feel proud of any of that. I guess I don't feel proud of much of anything. I don't even remember what I used to enjoy anymore. It's like I'm just going through the motions."

"That makes sense, Billy. You've been through a lot, and not just with the gremlins. It sounds like you had a lot of pressure from your parents to make money at home too: holding down a steady job while your dad worked on his 'inventions.' It's almost like you had to be the grown-up in your house. That can cause a lot of stress."

Billy sits with this for a moment. "Yeah, I guess I was asked to do a lot by my folks. And now I guess I feel like I'm being asked to do a lot by Kate too. And I feel responsible for Gizmo. He isn't just a pet; he's like my kid. So I went from parenting my parents to trying to be a provider for me and

Kate and now to parenting Gizmo. When do I get to just be a kid?" At this, Billy's lower lip begins to tremble.

In a compassionate yet firm voice we say, "But you aren't a kid anymore, Billy."

Softly, Billy begins to cry. "I worried so much all the time when I was growing up. Even before I knew what a job really was, I wanted one. I wanted to help my mom and my dad. By the time I was sixteen, I was working almost full time at the bank and helping out when I could at the Christmas-tree farm. Kate had it even worse than I did—she worked seven nights a week at the local bar!"

"It sounds like you got used to a high-stress way of life from a very young age."

"Yeah, and then Gizmo showed up, and then we had the gremlin infestation. And, honestly, being super on and aware really helped us survive the attack. I hoped things would calm down after Gizmo left, but I still felt keyed up and on edge. Kate and I moved to the city, hoping that would help. But it just got worse. I'm still not sleeping well. And now I think it might be something else."

"Something else? Can we ask, Billy, have you been feeling down? Like there's a boulder sitting on your chest and no matter what you do, you just can't seem to lift it?"

"Hey? How did you know that?" Billy asks as he wipes his eyes with an offered tissue.

"Billy, we've seen symptoms like this before. You've done amazing things in your life—faced off gremlins twice! But as a result of these struggles and being asked to take on more than you were capable of taking on as a child, you've inadvertently spawned some gremlins of your own: anxiety gremlins, to be precise. It sounds like they've been with you for years, and now, as a result, you've welcomed a new houseguest."

"Oh no . . . it's not the spider gremlin?!"

"The spider— No, Billy, we're talking about depression and anxiety."

"Wait, what?"

"Ironically enough, Billy, we like to think of anxiety in terms of gremlins. Think about it: symptoms of anxiety such as shallow breathing, rapid heart rate, racing thoughts, feeling on edge, and difficulty sleeping all happen when we are being attacked by gremlins."

Billy stares at us in amazement. "That is just like gremlins!"

"And just like Gizmo, each of us comes with some special self-care instructions, and when we don't or can't follow those, we spawn gremlins."

"Hmm, I think I get what you mean, but I'm not sure. Do you mean like how Kate always says that if she doesn't get her coffee first thing she can't function as a person?"

"Yes, exactly! You have self-care activities that would help you too, Billy. But it's possible no one helped you find out what they were. And this is where things get more complicated."

"Oh no."

"Oh yes. Sometimes, when we go too long trying to manage our anxiety gremlins on our own, the lazy houseguest depression moves in.[xxxiii] At first, he seems helpful. He tells us to relax and sit down on the sofa because nothing really matters anyway. But after a while, this message starts to bother us. There are things in our life we do like doing! We might even start to get bed sores. But depression persists, insisting that everything is worthless as he attempts to keep us sedentary and stuck."

Billy pauses and fidgets with his hoodie strings. "I have kind of been feeling like why worry; it doesn't do any good."

"Exactly! Billy, we think that the first step is learning how to parent yourself. What we mean by that is learning some of the self-care activities that you genuinely need to function. Can you think of any?"

"Well... this might sound kind of funny."

"We're ready to laugh."

"My parents almost always bought us soda to drink. But I don't think I like soda. I think I really like water."

We laugh. "Which is weird because Mogwai need to stay away from water?"

Billy smiles slowly. "Yeah."

[xxxiii] We felt that discussing Demogorgons after Billy's trauma would be too much, so we went with a friendlier image for him. Therapeutic Fanfiction—it's adaptable!

"Well, Billy, this is a great example of the idea that we each need different things to stay gremlin-free—or at least keep them contained in their wicker basket. It sounds like for you, more water does the trick."

"Do you think there are other things about myself that I can learn to do that will help keep the gremlins at bay, and maybe even make my lazy houseguest depression move out?"

"Absolutely, Billy."

FANFIC CASE STUDY QUESTIONS:
Getting Curious with Your Gremlins

* In what ways did Billy try to use his skills to help himself and his friends?
* How was Billy limited in his attempts to engage in healing and self-care by the systemic structures of his surroundings?
* What is the relationship between Billy's anxiety gremlins and his lazy houseguest, depression?

YOGA PRACTICE:
How to Calm Your Inner Gremlins

When we feel overrun with gremlins, it can be hard to focus. This yoga practice helps you to embody the act of placing the gremlins back in their baskets and finding your center once again. Remember to be mindful of your body and to make adjustments as needed. You can always wait for the gremlin to come to you.

1. Mountain Pose: Begin in a comfortable standing or seated position with your arms at your sides. Take a moment to simply observe the gremlins that are crawling around.

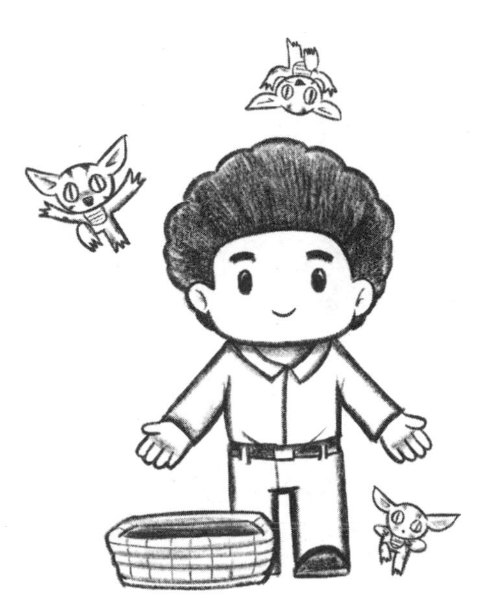

2. Upward Salute: Identify a particularly troublesome gremlin and reach up high to grab it.

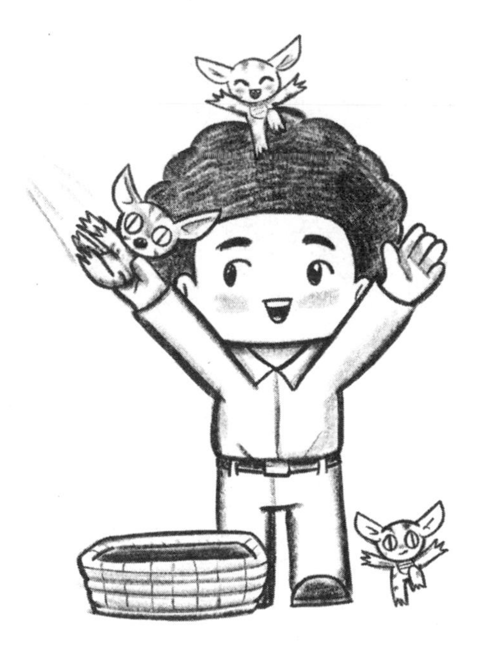

3. Standing Forward Bend: Fold the upper body forward and place the gremlin in its basket.

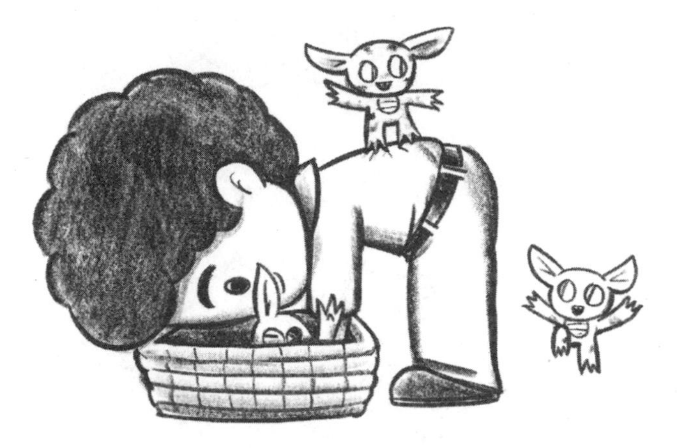

4. Halfway Lift: It will naturally crawl right out, so lift your upper body halfway to catch the little rascal.

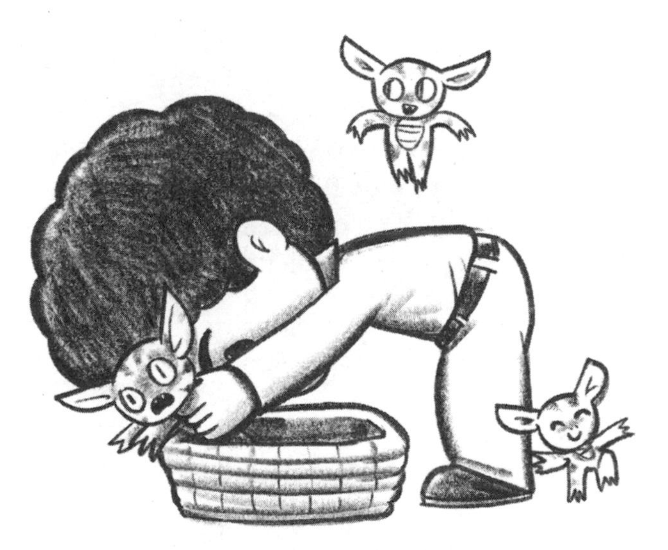

5. Standing Forward Bend: Fold forward again to place the gremlin in its basket.

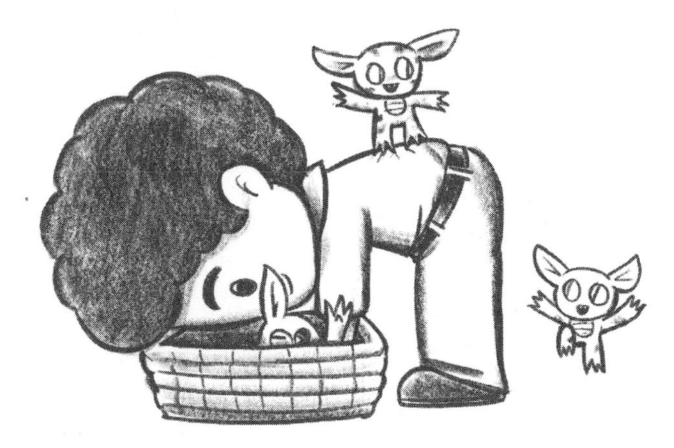

6. Upward Salute: Reach arms high up overhead again and repeat for all other gremlins that you find.

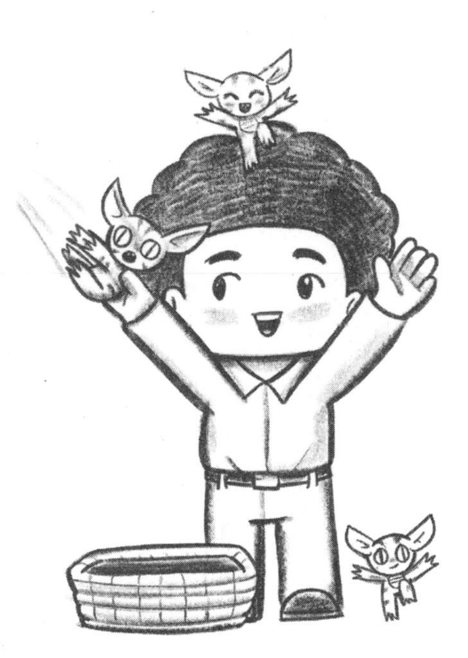

7. Hands to Heart Center: Once you are out of gremlins, bring your hands to your heart and allow yourself to feel gratitude for the work that you've done.

Resilience and Posttraumatic Growth through Fandoms

Magic doesn't come from talent; it comes from pain.

—ELIOT WAUGH, *THE MAGICIANS*, "THE SOURCE OF MAGIC"[89]

As practicing therapists, we have encountered the following request countless times: "Can you fix me?" Despite its frequency, the question always takes us by surprise. We respond with some version of the following: "You are neither broken nor flawed. And the idea that we have the ability to 'fix' anything about you, a fellow human on this great journey called life, implies that there is something innately 'wrong' with you and something innately 'right' about us, which we do not believe."

The idea that a person can or needs to be "fixed" bothers us because it presupposes a binary system of extremes. Some of the most common binaries we hear in our office are folks saying they feel like they are either good or bad, right or wrong, broken or fixed, and smart or dumb. In our experience, most of existence sits somewhere on a spectrum between two polarities; a wizard arrives precisely when he means to, after all. Or, to put it another way, we believe that we exist in shades of (Gandalf the) gray.[90]

Shittily Wrapped Gifts

The shittily wrapped gift (yes, we absolutely use this language in therapy sessions) is a terrifically useful gift that can be yours forever once you remove the awful packaging. What might this look like IRL? Perhaps you'd like more confidence in daily life because it will help you compassionately hold your ground when you ask for a raise in your yearly review, which no doubt was delayed by at least two months because Bob in HR is super busy. (We're all busy, Bob.) But to get this confidence, you're going to have to practice. For example, when you're given the task of presenting at all board meetings for the next two months, that's the shitty packaging in action! With each presentation, you've removed one layer of awful wrapping paper and are one step closer to self-confidence! If you were in therapy with us, we might say, "Look at this amazing opportunity you've been given to practice new skills and gain confidence on your hero's journey!" At that point, you might feel more like throwing the stuffed Mordin plushie at us than heeding the call to adventure.

Shittily wrapped gifts come in all shapes and sizes. Sometimes, they are even bite-sized. You've probably had an experience in which a close friend or partner reflected a hard message or painful truth. "You hurt my feelings when you were late for the movie. Seeing the previews for the next MCU movie is really important to me." "You promised you'd take the trash out this week, but you forgot again. I don't want to be in the position of micromanaging, but what do I do when I remember and you don't?"

Accepting hard truths about our current behavior can be some of the smelliest types of shittily wrapped gifts. But they offer us a powerful opportunity to reflect on our habits and make changes that help both ourselves and those around us.

Truth is tricky. When given from a place of emotional vulnerability, it holds the opportunity for growth and change. But when we give the gift of truth with insults and criticism, it's like taking a shittily wrapped gift and wrapping it in barbed wire. We'll get into this more in chapter 7. For now, let's focus on the idea that ugly wrapping paper can hold a great gift inside. You might need some help unwrapping the gift. Better to ask for help than attain your gift along with 1,001 paper cuts.

Resilience

Rather than thinking of growth and change in terms of fixing, we recommend conceiving of it in terms of healing. Healing is a complex circular process that allows for the reality that discomfort and even pain are sometimes necessary to "get better," or, in other words, recover. The fix-it approach views people as equivalent to their problems, whereas healing sees a person in relationship to their problems. Healing offers the perspective that a creature, situation, or an event can contain multitudes. Recall from up top the confidence example. A fix-it approach equates self-doubt or insecurity with a flaw in the person and seeks to alter both the person and the behavior. Did you ever "should" yourself into a bad mood? "I should have washed the dishes sooner, I should have exercised this morning, I should have caught the earlier bus." We often say to irritated clients, "Stop shoulding on yourself!" The fix-it shoulds shackle us to the problem and intensify feelings of disappointment, sadness, worry, and dread. The healing approach acknowledges that you are doing your best; you just might need some new tools to help you on your hero's journey.

Resilience[91] is a healing tool often used interchangeably with the posttraumatic growth tool (don't worry, we'll get there),[92] but it has some key differences. Both tools can help you tackle a difficult quest. Resilience offers the ability to return to baseline after the quest is over.[93] Think Cyclops from nearly every iteration of the *X-Men*. Part of what makes Cyclops insufferable to some folks is that although he fights valiantly and does his best to lead the team the way Professor X envisions, he doesn't change a whole lot from quest to quest.[94] Certainly, there are some exceptions—*The Age of Apocalypse*[95] and the *Cable* comic book[96] arcs being perhaps the best examples of Cyclops as a growing and shifting character—but most of the time Cyclops is able to use resilience to fight a tough battle with Magneto and return to the X-Jet with his ego intact. When he encounters an obstacle, he bounces back, returning to the same ol' lovable four eyes. Resilience denotes a person's innate ability to deal with difficult situations and rebound from them. Folks sometimes think of resilience as being inborn, almost like destiny. In other words, you're born with your allotted soup container of resilience, and when it's depleted that means no more resilience for you. In this interpretation, resilience seems to function like Link's fairy bottles in a boss fight.

While we respect everyone's right to form an opinion, this particular representation of resilience doesn't really speak to us, in part because recent anecdotal and quantitative research seems to indicate that human beings have a lot more control over their resilience than first thought.[97] Rather than predestined fairy bottles, it might be most helpful to think of resilience as a resilience stamina bar with a storage level that can increase or decrease depending on how we treat ourselves or how we are treated by other beings in close proximity to us.[98] In chapter 3, we talked about the importance of self-care related to minimizing or downright exterminating anxiety gremlins. The concept for resilience is similar, with the addition that the size of our resilience bar seems to be determined somewhat by how we are treated as children.[99]

The way in which we are cared for when we are young Baby Yodas influences us a whole lot. It even influences how our genes express themselves![xxxiv] For those unfamiliar with the Baby Yoda memes and GIFs that swept the nation in 2019–2020, we really encourage you to give this creature a hearty google. Because Baby Yoda is the cutest—though, technically, the moniker "Baby Yoda" is a nickname given by the fans. Baby Yoda, known first as the Child and then later as Grogu in *The Mandalorian* TV series, is not, in fact, original Yoda's relative.[100] In season 1, Baby Yoda is found by the Mandalorian, also referred to as Mando, a bounty hunter who initially plans to turn Baby Yoda over to some sketchy Sithy sympathizers, but then he has a change of heart! Mando looks deep into Baby Yoda's eyes and sees an innocent life, triggering memories of his own war-torn childhood and the Mandalorian people who adopted and cared for him when he was just a little older than Baby Yoda. Together, Mando and Baby Yoda explore the galaxy, making friends with Gina Carano and Carl Weathers along the way. Really, if you haven't watched the show, we encourage you to give it a watch. It even has Taika Waititi as a fun (with a death complex) droid!

[xxxiv] We are referring to epigenetics or changes in a gene's phenotype. Basically, certain genes turn certain genetic traits on or off, based on the external environment.

Back to the resilience stamina bar, research suggests that our core caregivers—parents, grandparents, teachers, cousins—determine the size of our stamina bar[xxxv] based on how they treat us during the early milestones of childhood. This lines up with attachment theory, a process initially researched by John Bowlby and Mary Ainsworth that seeks to describe the early interactional patterns between a child and their core caregiver(s) that teach the child how to emotionally connect with other living beings.[101] These early relationships help the child to grow their resilience stamina bar. So, the more loving, compassionate, and secure interactions a child has when they are young (think ages zero to three), the longer the resilience stamina bar gets. But what about kids who don't have consistent and loving interactions with their core caregivers? Are they just doomed to have baby bars?

Well, yes and no. One of the things that has baffled psychology for decades is the fact that some children who have just the worst homelife—we're talking about Baby Yodas who never had a Mando to save them and were instead surrounded by shady Sithy sympathizers or sometimes straight-up Sith warriors—demonstrate a fuckton of resilience. How can this be? We posit that the unique outcome has to do with that other tool we mentioned: posttraumatic growth. The other issue at play here is fandom attachment.

Yes, IRL parents are important. Despite what Langston Hughes said about how children should be born without them,[xxxvi] we won't fly in the face of decades of research supporting the importance of core caregivers.[102] But we will formally request that the definition of that term be broadened to include fandom attachment. Recall that fandom attachment is the one-way relationship between you and a beloved fictional character or the persona of a public figure.[xxxvii]

Let's get on the trolly to the neighborhood of make-believe and look at some childhood examples. When you were Baby Yoda, did you ever watch

[xxxv] Or stamina wheel, depending on what video game you're playing.

[xxxvi] No, seriously, he actually said that.

[xxxvii] For the Jungians in the room, we are referring to the character-created public figures like Paris Hilton or Kim Kardashian as opposed to the Jungian archetype of the persona. In some cases, these two concepts are linked; it might be most helpful to think of them as two semi-overlapping circles in a Venn diagram.

Mister Rogers' Neighborhood and weep every time Mr. Rogers looked into the camera and into your heart and said, "You're special just the way you are"?[103] No? Maybe that was just us, then. Even if you didn't sob like us, you probably felt warm and safe and seen. Or perhaps your fandom of choice back in the day was *The Magic School Bus*—a fun show based on an acid trip for the whole fam! *Chip 'n' Dale: Rescue Rangers*? *Dragon Tales*? *Care Bears*? *Star Trek: The Next Generation*?[104] *Reading Rainbow*? *Doctor Who*? If you don't see your childhood fandom of choice here, write it in (or type it in if you're reading via screen). These early and loving fandom attachments are just as much a part of your experience as your IRL attachments. When you co-created a story in which Counselor Troi told you that you're a worthy person or an imagined being encouraged by Ms. Frizzle or saw yourself being read to by Geordi La Forge, who inexplicably had functioning eyes in the daytime, then you experienced the power of childhood fandom attachment to nurture you. And as you co-created this world of loving imagined characters, your resilience bar started to grow! Positive relationships are healing, regardless of type. And research shows that it only takes one positive adult figure in a child's life to aid in resilience; why can't that person be a character?[105]

We must acknowledge that this field of research is still quite young. And, we'd argue, it has been held back due to unfair prejudice in the medical and psychological communities against video games and movie or television characters. Reading has long been accepted as beneficial to developing minds and empathic hearts. Though some of our colleagues might disagree, we posit that fandom attachment transcends its medium in terms of healing powers. We also very gently offer that gaming is a co-creative experience very similar to reading that, in some ways, surpasses reading in the ways it allows for the creation of worlds.[106] *Minecraft and Animal Crossing,* anyone? We are definitely not hating on reading—clearly, we are pro the written word—but we defend and extol the healing powers of fandom attachment in all its myriad forms.

Posttraumatic Growth

Okay, mutants, let's jump back to *X-Men* for this conversation. For those of you unfamiliar with the *X-Men,* this is a term of loving endearment. *Mutant,* in the context of the X-Men comic universe, denotes a human being blessed with a genetic gift that gives special power. Storm's mutant genes give her the power to control the weather. Cyclops's mutant genes give him optic lasers that shoot out of his eyeballs. Jean Grey, aka Marvel Girl, aka Phoenix's mutant genes give her both telepathic and telekinetic abilities. We love all the *X-Men* characters, but for our purposes in this chapter we are going to focus on Storm.

Like many X-Men (and frankly like many of us), Storm had a tough childhood. Though things start off seemingly bright with two parents, one of whom is a kick-ass sorceress, Storm's happy home life is short-lived: orphaned at six years old in the violence of the Arab-Israeli war,[xxxviii] baby Storm wanders the streets of Cairo.[107] With no Mando in sight, Storm has to make her own way. She joins a gang of kid grifters and survives as a thief. Now some of you might think, *Hey, Achmed el-Gibar, leader of the kid grifter gang, was kinda like Mando!* We encourage you to take another look at that idea. One of the defining traits of the Baby Yoda and Mando dynamic is that Mando does not ask Baby Yoda to ever use their[xxxix] powers to get them out of tight situations. Nor does he ever exploit Baby Yoda's gifts for his own gain. Carl Weathers asks this of Baby Yoda, and it is laughed off by the rest of the team because, duh, Baby Yoda is a baby. It is not appropriate to give Baby Yoda the role of the warrior yet. Storm's new parental figure takes the opposite approach: Achmed el-Gibar uses children for his own capital gain. Life for Storm continues to be, well, stormy (we had to), though there are some bright spots that include a meet-cute with her once and future Charles Xavier.[108] But, all in all, life stays tough for Storm until her teenage years when she joins up with a tribe of the Serengeti, taking on the role of the weather goddess. Things take a still more positive turn for Storm when Charles Xavier[xl] returns and invites her to join the X-Men.[109]

[xxxviii] It is also known as the Suez Crisis, which, yes, is a real thing. X-Men was ripping from the headlines before *Law & Order* made it a cliché.

[xxxix] While we acknowledge that Baby Yoda's creator, Jon Favreau, assigns masculine pronouns to Baby Yoda, we couldn't nope that harder if we tried. It's the future, Jon; we've transcended binary gender as a meaningful construct.

[xl] He was busy training other mutant kids and fighting off the Shadow King and also maybe siring David Holler, aka Legion. As with most things in Marvel comic books, things get a lot more confusing, and nothing totally fits together. But, hey, that's what happens when a story lasts for decades and has hundreds of writers!

That was a lot of back story. But what does it all mean? If we look closely, we can see the makings of posttraumatic growth for Storm. Post-traumatic growth is a process by which a person heals and grows through their trauma.[110] A person doesn't bounce back to baseline like in resilience. Rather, their painful circumstances are part of what helps them to transcend old behaviors, break away from outdated modes of thought, and gain new skills.[111] This might sound familiar, and, if it does, that's great work—you're paying attention! Posttraumatic growth *is* a type of hero's journey.

In order for a person to complete the hero's journey of posttraumatic growth rather than get stuck at posttraumatic stress disorder (PTSD), they need supportive community; a clear sense of purpose, that is, a meaning for their suffering; and time to reflect on their pain. Perhaps you were about to point out that Storm absolutely suffers from PTSD[xli] as a result of nearly being buried alive.[xlii] We agree that Storm certainly struggles with PTSD.[112] Most of the mutants in the X-Men's reality struggle with trauma to greater or lesser degrees. Being a mutant—a minority—can be extremely marginalizing. Here is where the tool, or, more aptly, the journey, of posttraumatic growth can help you and every mutant to heal. For now, let's return to Storm.

It seems pretty clear that Storm has a decent-sized resilience bar: Though losing her parents was awful, they really seemed to love and care about her, which no doubt resulted in some secure attachment. Secure attachment happens when a child can rely on the loving support and structure of their core caregivers, helping them to detach when one or more of the caregivers leave and reattach when they return.[113] Storm's ability to seek new community with varying degrees of support and to detach when they leave or when they no longer support her indicates that she has the tool of secure attachment. Thus, she also can access supportive community, a key component of the posttraumatic growth journey. Storm has a propensity for reflection. She's often found sitting on the Xavier mansion's roof, either processing her

---

[xli] Can PTSD and PTG exist in the same human . . . er, mutant? Maybe! Scholars can't agree.

[xlii] In the comics, she is described as having claustrophobia. And while we agree that she certainly meets full criteria for claustrophobia, we're confident that PTSD is the underlying issue, with claustrophobia functioning as a symptom of her PTSD.

feelings or helping her good friend Wolverine sort through his. This natural inclination for reflection, coupled with the supportive teammates she finds with the X-Men, enables her to continue on her journey.

But Storm fully begins to heal when she finds purpose. Life on the streets stunted her growth and no doubt exacerbated the PTSD she would later struggle to overcome when she joined the X-Men. Storm finds purpose[114] as the weather goddess of the Serengeti tribe, but she is also separate from her new adopted community who put her on a pedestal because, well, they see her as the weather goddess. When Xavier finds her and pitches her the idea of joining his team, Storm sees the chance to find community and time for reflection and to lead a life of purpose. While the healing journey is never easy for Storm, nor is it for any of us, she continues to evolve and grow as part of the X-Men. Eventually, Storm turns her pain into emotional strength, gaining deeper understanding and compassion for herself, her fellow mutants, and humans.

One of the key ways you can learn how to grow through trauma is through meaning-making by engaging with stories as listener, speaker, and/or creator. Examples of fandom characters who have both healed and grown from trauma are Sansa, Missandei, and Daenerys of *Game of Thrones*,[115] as well as Buffy of *Buffy the Vampire Slayer*,[116] Zelda of *The Legend of Zelda* video game series, and Geralt, Yennefer, and Ciri of *The Witcher* video game series.[117] Early anecdotal research suggests playing video games that incorporate elements of posttraumatic growth into gameplay can aid and potentially catalyze healing for gamers.[118] We will go into further detail on meaning in the next chapter, but we want to take this opportunity to name-drop one of our favorite thinkers on the power of meaning: Viktor Frankl. A survivor of the Holocaust, Frankl wrote the book *Man's Search for Meaning,* in which he explores the healing power of choice.[119] In short, we can't choose our circumstances, but we can choose how we react to those circumstances and ultimately make meaning from them.

In our therapeutic work, we encourage clients to bring fandoms into session so we can help them explore and understand how, for example, Yennefer's journey to self-actualize, that is, attain her own independent identity, mirrors the clients' current journey to become a separate individual from their family of origin and embrace the values and beliefs that resonate with them.[120] A necessary component for posttraumatic growth is having a narrative framework to understand its meaning. If pain is simply a byproduct of an unfeeling universe, we are more likely to get stuck in the abyss of despair. In the video game series *The Legend of Zelda,* part of what helps Link grow from his trauma is the belief that he is the hero of Hyrule.[121] He both is chosen and chooses to save his community.

It's no accident, then, that the game in which Link struggles the most with the symptoms of PTSD—depression, confusion, memory loss, and flashbacks—is *Majora's Mask.* Here, Link finds himself in Termina instead of Hyrule and is thus no longer the hero.[122] Without the protective meaning of his hero's journey, Link struggles like never before to forge connections with strangers, make progress (the only way to make progress in the game is to reset it before the world ends), and experience joy.[123] Therapeutic Fanfiction helps an individual to find within their fandoms of choice a blueprint to use to create their own meaningful narrative. Ultimately, the universe might be uncaring. But that doesn't mean you have to be apathetic toward yourself. You and the community you choose can create, grow, and sustain the meaning of your life.

Before we wrap up this chapter, let's look at one last example of the ways engaging with fandom fosters healing. One of the most popular indie games in recent memory, *Journey*, has been cited by numerous gamers as helping them to process their pain and heal from challenging experiences.[124] *Journey* is the hero's journey or monomyth brought to life in its purest form. In the game, your avatar is a genderless hero who explores the citadels of a mountain range. As you climb, you encounter archetypal images, such as the mother goddess, the trickster, the child, and the father, in addition to other similarly robed genderless figures like yourself. In his *The Masks of God* multivolume work, Joseph Campbell describes many types of initiation rites practiced in cultures around the globe meant to simulate the hero's journey. These rites symbolized an individual's transition from childhood into adulthood and provided a testing ground where they learned how to enact the hero's journey in their own life.[125] Video games like *Journey* can serve a similar purpose to these early initiation rites, equipping gamers with both the tools and language to understand their struggles and make meaning from them.

FANFIC CASE STUDY:
X-Men, Weathering the Storm

Following a frenetic stint in the city that never sleeps and is occasionally overrun with gremlins, we decided to take up offices in more relaxed environs, the picturesque small town of North Salem, New York. For the first several months, business was slow, and we found ourselves with ample time to relax in each of our preferred modes—reading Russian novels for Spock and daytime catnaps for Kirk. One slow-moving Wednesday, we look up from our respective desks as heavy clouds move across the sky. "Looks like rain. And how odd—sunny skies were forecast all week." As a flash of lightning cut across the now dark sky, we turn toward a wind in the door and a soft rap of knuckles on our office door frame.

"The doctors Therapise, I presume?" Her deep and resonant voice sweeps through our office just like the wind that preceded her.

"Storm? Or, should we say, Ororo Munroe?" We ask, rising to usher her in.

"I can see my reputation precedes me."

"Indeed. We must remind you, though, that we are not doctors per se but trained and highly skilled marriage and family therapists."

With a slight wave (that, incidentally, exactly coincides with another shock of lightning), she declines the tea we offer, leaning back into the sofa cushions. "Names need not be exact to apply."

We let this go for now, making a mental note to circle back with a clarifying question later, as we take careful notice of the way the weather outside mirrors almost down to the moment the shifts in Ororo's facial expressions.

"You remind me of the professor. He, too, kept many things to himself."

"Our apologies. We were just noticing the relationship between your physical movements and—"

"The weather outside? Yes, I've gotten much better at controlling my powers. Panic attacks that used to cause tornadoes that ripped through towns are now—"

"Gentle lightning storms?"

Ororo chuckles—her first smile of the session—and shrugs. The darkening clouds outside shift from navy to gray. "Maybe I will take that cup of tea, and cream and sugar if you have it—the English way, old habits from Xavier's school for gifted youngsters."

"Was the professor English?" we ask, passing her the sugar bowl.

"Indeed. Oxford trained. He had some of the colonial problems that come from such an education, but a compassionate heart makes up for many flaws."

"It sounds like you see the best in people."

"Sometimes. It wasn't always this way for me. I grew up on the streets of Cairo taking advantage of people's kindness—a pickpocket," Storm turns her spoon slowly in her tea, clouds of cream ballooning up around the handle. "I don't even remember my parents. The professor offered to retrieve the memories for me, but I never liked his habit of poking around in people's heads without permission."

"He didn't always check for consent?"

"No." Outside, rain begins to fall.

"What brings you to our offices, Storm?"

"Ororo, please."

"We must admit we'd gathered from the news that you were on hiatus from the X-Men."

"Yes, I was working on my marriage with T'Challa, Black Panther. Perhaps if I'd come to you sooner things would have turned out differently. But that's all over now."

"The marriage or the hiatus?"

Ororo smiles ruefully. "Both. Well, I'd like to return to the X-Men, take up the mantle of leadership. But I'm concerned . . . I haven't been myself recently." She notices our glance to the window.

"Oh, it's not that." She waves her hand and suddenly the rain ceases, clouds disperse, and sunlight streams in, glaring off the glass coffee table so brightly that we see stars. "My control is fine. Better than it ever was. It's just . . . I've been feeling disquieted."

"Unhappy?" we offer.

"Not exactly, just . . ." Storm pauses and for the first time looks out the window. She whispers softly, "I'm afraid to go back to the school. I'm afraid I'm not a very good leader."

Hundreds of examples to the contrary aside, we sit in silence with Ororo, watching her watch the weather outside.

"The professor was a good if flawed teacher. Scott and I worked well together, for the most part. Even El-Gibar, leader of our band of thieves, was firm but kind."

"How old were you when you joined the thieves?"

"Six. But I was by no means the youngest."

"Were there any adults in the gang?"

"I didn't say he was perfect; I just said he had things to share too—useful teachings."

"And we don't disagree. But we would point out that you are showing compassion for each of your mentors, including El-Gibar, who trained children as thieves and took a cut of their profits. What would it be like to extend that compassion to yourself?"

"Every team I've led, I've failed. The Morlocks, both Callisto[126] and Marrow,[127] counted on me to help them, and I didn't. I thought they needed a place amongst the X-Men, like I did. I didn't bother to consider that they might have wanted a different life. I didn't even ask. I treat leadership too much like being a goddess—always assuming I know best. Or like the Weather Witch—that's how Gambit used to tease me. I used to take it so personally. Now, I wonder if he wasn't just trying to bring me back down to earth."

"Being vulnerable is human, Ororo."

"Yes, but I'm a mutant."

"What do these different names mean to you?"

Storm raises one white eyebrow.

"Mutant. Human. Storm. Ororo. Rain Goddess. Weather Witch. You mentioned earlier that names need not be exact to apply. And, yet, you corrected us when we called you Storm."

"I thought my human name would be better here."

"Your mutant name?"

She smiles then. "You're as good as Arya said you were—though not half as witty."

"We'll take the compliment."

"You have a point, perhaps. I have had many names."

"You've had many roles. Do you have a favorite?"

"Name or role?"

"Either."

Storm opens her mouth as if to speak, then, changing her mind, takes another sip of tea and stares out the window. The clouds reappear and shift, a cumulus half obscuring the sun. "If I'm honest, it's still the Weather Witch that comes to mind, the goddess. After all these years, she's the part my heart goes back to. Ainet, my adopted mother, loved me—but always at a distance. I think even she believed I was the goddess foretold and not just a little girl, orphaned by war—just another human like all the rest." She glances at us. "Yes, perhaps the names aren't so important."

"Ororo, it makes sense that you held onto the role of goddess; it saved you. It gave you your first real family after the death of your parents. But it might not be the role that fits you best anymore. It might be time to write a new story, find new meaning."

"New meaning in what?"

A low rumble of thunder sounds. "Meaning in being Storm. And Ororo. Mutant and Human. With the power of a goddess. Maybe you don't have to choose. Maybe there's a way to integrate them all."

"I contain many parts."

We smile. "Don't we all?"

FANFIC CASE STUDY QUESTIONS:
Tracking the Storm

* Identify the helpers that Storm has in her life. How did they help her to both heal and grow through her trauma?

- Now think about some of the important people and fandom characters in your life. List their names and the ways you could lean on them for support, care, and compassion.
- The roles of goddess, member of the X-Men, and team leader help Storm make meaning in her life. What are the roles in your life that help you to make meaning?

A MEDITATION ON LOVING KINDNESS[128]

May all mutants everywhere be happy and free.

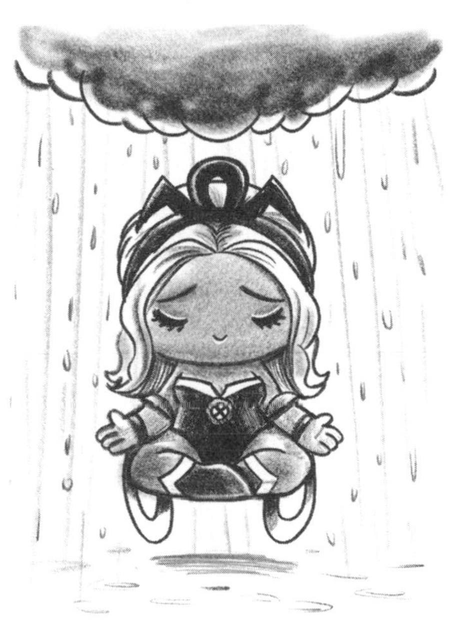

Today, we are going to practice a variant of the loving-kindness meditation. The loving-kindness meditation is an ancient practice centered around the idea that all people and, in fact, all beings are worthy of unconditional acceptance, warmth, and love. Today, we will focus our loving-kindness practice on extending this gift of unconditional love, acceptance, and support to ourselves and to all creatures—mutant and human alike.

You may want to start this meditation reclining, sitting, or, in honor of the weather goddess herself, outside. We encourage you to take whatever posture is most comfortable to you and to shift your focus to your breathing. Take a full deep breath in and a full exhale out. Let the corners of your eyes relax, and let your gaze soften. Remember that whether you identify as a mutant, human, superhero, or witch, all of you are welcome here.

Picture yourself or a past version of you in your mind's eye. Perhaps a childhood iteration of yourself, full of play and mirth. Or a young adult you, full of strength and conviction. Notice how you feel toward this version of you; without any judgment, just notice. No matter what the answer is, could you offer this version of you some compassion for what they're going through right now? Take a moment and send out this message of loving kindness to this you:

May you be well.

May you be peaceful.

May you be kind.

Take a deep breath in and a breath out.

Shift your attention to a person, animal, or character who is important to you. Perhaps you imagine a close personal friend such as T'Challa, the Black Panther. Or perhaps you picture a family member, Rogue or Wolverine. Picture this being clearly in your mind's eye. Notice how you feel toward this being; without any judgment, just notice. No matter what the answer is, could you offer this version of you some compassion for what they're going through right now? Take a moment and extend this message of loving kindness:

May you be well.

May you be peaceful.

May you be kind.

Take a deep breath in and a deep breath out.

Now, invite your intention inward to rest on a person, animal, or character whom you find challenging in your present life. Perhaps you picture Magneto, or perhaps Mystique, the mother who both loves and hurts. Notice how you feel toward this being; without any judgment, just notice. No matter what the answer is, could you offer this individual compassion for what they may be going through right now? Take a moment and extend a message of loving kindness:

May you be well.

May you be peaceful.

May you be kind.

Finally, shift your attention to yourself just as you are. Notice how you feel toward yourself; without any judgment, just notice. No matter what the answer is, could you offer yourself compassion for what you are going through right now? Take a moment and extend this message of loving kindness:

May I be well.

May I be peaceful.

May I be kind.

Take a deep breath in and a deep breath out. Bring attention back to your physical body. Whenever you are ready, return to the space you are in.

5

Writing Therapeutic Fanfiction

We each gave the other a beautiful gift. A choice.
We are the authors of our stories now.

—DOLORES ABERNATHY, *WESTWORLD*, "THE PASSENGER"[129]

Humans have been writing fanfiction since quite literally the dawn of time. And, no, we're not just referring to that scene with the apes and the bones from *2001: A Space Odyssey,* which is a riff on Homer's the *Odyssey*. Charles Dickens's *A Christmas Carol,* William Shakespeare's *Romeo and Juliet,* Jane Austen's *Emma*, and Sir Arthur Conan Doyle's *Sherlock Holmes*, and basically every musical production ever, are examples of the many stories that gave birth to fanfiction adaptations written, shared, and rewritten throughout human civilization. In America, writers like Langston Hughes and Zora Neale Hurston reestablished a place for Black voices and stories within the dominant white and European spaces of early twentieth-century America. Hurston's entire oeuvre can be understood as a synthesis and rebirth of African America folklore and tales,[130] i.e., myths.[xliii]

[xliii] Recent accusations of embellishment or downright forgery do not diminish Hurston's work, but rather offer a fanfiction dimension to her novels and anthologies.

Sometimes the fanfic even stars an adorable terrier: What's the story, Wishbone?[131] What all of these stories have in common is that they asked the question "what if?" What if Sherlock and John were a definitely, but not canonically, gay couple in modern London? What if a bunch of stories featured a Jack Russell terrier protagonist? And the answer, my friends, is that they would be better—or, at the very least, more diverse in their scope, vision, and reach. Fanfiction asks the question "what if" and then answers with varying degrees of success.

When we talk about Therapeutic Fanfiction, we are talking about doing the very same thing with our own lives: What if I changed careers? What if I dated this person instead? Or what if I loved myself authentically exactly as I am? What would that story look like? And it helps us to answer these questions using the power of myth. Mythology contains the archetypes that allow us to tap into the primal power of play. As Joseph Campbell once theorized, human beings are special not because of our tools but because of our imaginations. He believed that our naked faces (read, nonhairy mammal faces) gave us the power like never before to communicate and understand a wide range of emotions and ideas.[132] Why are we born as such helpless li'l babies?

Campbell theorized that this all goes back to the malleability of the brain. The less developed a brain at birth, the more capability a species has to respond and make changes based on their environment. Although science still has a ways to go to verify the following claim, Campbell went one step further—because, really, why not?—and postulated that all earth creatures are born with presets or schemas that help them understand and respond to their environment. There's actually scientific evidence for this.[133] But the next bit is where things get debatable: Campbell took Jung's idea about the collective unconscious and thought, *What if every creature had access to the collective unconscious, and some species are just more separate from it than others?* Does that sound weird? Well, welcome to existential mythology, friends. It's measured in Jeremy Bearamies.[xliv] So to wrap up, humans are special because we are emotionally sensitive beings who have access to both the collective unconscious that might contain all the knowledge of

[xliv] Shout out to *The Good Place*.

Earth and the ability via personal consciousness and unconscious to create new knowledge and new actions. How do we create this newness? Play!

If you thought play was just for kids and not really all that important, well, your naked face would disagree. The idea that play is only for children is a Westworld Construct that we heartily encourage you to question. We invite you to look around at all the ways that you already play and how that play makes your world an even better place. We would imagine, friend, that you actually engage in a lot of play if you've picked up this book. But you might be new to the particular play of fanfiction.

Fanfic!

Fanfiction is founded on the practice of rejecting those narratives or stories that are out of character for fandom favorites and creating stories that are more truly resonant. Fanfiction in daily life allows fans to break out of the stories that no longer serve them and create those that empower them.[134] *Star Trek* is considered the birth fandom of fanfic. Back when the Enterprise was first flying, a group of (mostly women) thinkers began to concoct their own stories about their beloved crew. And Gene Roddenberry[135] was fucking into it![xlv] Sherlock Holmes also has an incredibly long fanfic history. Sir Arthur was pretty chill about this as well.[136] The thing is, creators didn't get super elitist about owning characters until much later. Just try to slip in some Armand and Louis fanfic, and Anne Rice will have you sent to a metaphorical dungeon.[xlvi] Luckily, fanfiction is now a beloved outlet for fans, and there are safe spaces for writing, sharing, and offering feedback on each other's fic, such as Archive of Our Own, or AO3. There's fanfic for everything. Do you ship Neil Armstrong with Elon Musk?[xlvii] There's fic for that! Of course, what we just described is real person fic or RPF, which is considered taboo in some circles. We don't judge. We actually think that RPF is

[xlv] So maybe he just turned a blind eye to it. But in our headcanon, he was *into* it!

[xlvi] In case you weren't a teenager in the 1990s, Armand and Louis are characters from Anne Rice's *Interview with the Vampire*: #loveneverdies.

[xlvii] This is a real person fic on Archive of Our Own. Search as you must.

great because that's sort of the basis of Therapeutic Fanfiction. You are the real person who you are ficcing. This is your life, and you get to decide when the writers are going in the wrong direction and start to course-correct.

Just like Anne Rice,[137] there might be people in your life who don't like the new direction where you're taking your character, and that's okay. It isn't their story; it's yours. So you can thank Anne for her contribution to your story thus far and get down to the business of uniting Louis and Armand.[138] Or if you're thinking about ficcing your real life, you might thank your dear Aunt Anne, or your Aunt J.K. for that matter, for her contribution in raising you while compassionately letting her know that you are passing back all that anti-queer and anti-trans rhetoric she spoon-fed you with creamed corn, thankyouverymuch.

Step by Step, Day by Day

So far in this book, we have explored different aspects of the Therapeutic Fanfiction model: the hero's journey, fandom attachments, the Westworld Construct, externalization, personification, resilience, and posttraumatic growth. In upcoming chapters, we'll explore even more tools to add to your Therapeutic Fanfiction tool kit. Each question that you've asked yourself and asked about the world will help you with rewriting the story of your life. But how do you start the rewrite process? It's like they said on ABC's TGIF lineup: the journey of a thousand miles begins with one step—or something like that. The most important first step of Therapeutic Fanfiction is best symbolized by the archetype of the fellowship. Yes, that fellowship! We're talking *Lord of the Rings*'s Gandalf, Frodo, Sam, Meri, Pippin, Aragorn, Gimli, Legolas, and Boromir. Sigh, yes, even you Boromir, because everyone deserves the chance for love and redemption. This technique is a riff on a narrative therapy technique called re-membering. (It's not remembering; it's re-membering.)[139] It invites you to take stock of the people in your life and consider whom you experience as supportive and whom you experience as, well, unhelpful. Then you get to decide who gets invited inside your house and who needs to stay on the porch. Don't worry; this will make more sense in chapter 7 when we discuss rules, roles, and boundaries. Readers, join us, the writers, on an adventure to find our fellowship! We are creating the members who will help us during a particular quest, understanding that we can re-member at any time as the quest needs arise.

Whereas White and Epston envision re-membering as a stage that happens roughly midway through the therapeutic process and means changing your lineup of supportive friends and community, the fellowship step happens first and is more focused on rallying your fandom attachments. You can certainly include IRL folks in your fellowship, be they currently with you on this mortal plane or be they dead. The key is to mentally gather and then possibly physically write down (or type down) a list of fandom attachments, IRL attachments, and beloved fandom tools. You could also totally make a fellowship vision board. The guiding principle for who and what you choose are those characters, attributes, and tools that are in alignment with your personal goals and values. We chose the fellowship in this example because it embodies a group of friends embarking on a perilous quest—which is how we envision ourselves with you, reader. This fandom archetype aligns with our value of friendship and our goal to make the journey together.

Now we need to know what this quest is about. We have our mission statement: rewrite your story. But to do that we need to figure out the challenges that you and your fellowship are up against. Think back to chapter 3. Conjure forth the image of a depression Demogorgon and an anxiety gremlin. Terrifying, aren't they? But be not afraid! Remember that you have an entire list or vision board of the fandom fellowship here to help you on this quest! Maybe your challenges are best exemplified as No-Face, aka social anxiety. Perhaps your current struggle is with your family of origin (more on this in chapters 7 and 8). Make a list—or if you want, a shadow vision board—of these challenges. Set your lists or vision boards up side by side and try to match up the dyadic pairs. What do we mean by that? Well, Campbell and Jung had this idea that all mythic constructs came in pairs: Harry and Voldemort, Link and Shadow Link, Luke and Darth Vader, Black Panther and Killmonger, Storm and Callisto, and Buffy and Faith. Matching up your pairs will help you to map out the fandom attachments or tools that will help you on different parts of your journey.

Let's say that you have the Scooby gang from *Buffy the Vampire Slayer* on your vision board and you have anxiety gremlins on your shadow board.

The gremlins get the most activated for you around interactions with your overbearing boss. Before you match up, consider what it is about your boss that has the gremlins so activated. Is there an internal narrative you believe about yourself that your boss reinforces? Perhaps your boss confirms your strongly held belief that you are not good enough. How does this narrative serve you? Does it in fact harm you? Then it might be time for the power of fanfiction to change this story.

You might match Buffy up with your boss who intimidates you because you believe that you are a meek human, but you wish that you had more confidence. Buffy has a snarky confidence that feels like just the light you need against the shadow of your boss, whom you find humorless and stern. Or you might pair Willow with the gremlin that represents your relationship with a loved one because you've seen how she was able to work through many different difficult relationships with her own friends. If you don't find a match between the two boards or lists, take a moment and brainstorm a few more helpers for your fellowship. There are no rules for how many folks you can have. It's infinite! The most important thing is that your fellowship makes sense to you.

Once you've identified the dyads, you will be able to call upon your fandom attachment whenever you need them. So if your boss is being especially stern, you might notice that your internal monologue begins again about how you just aren't very good at anything, etc. Would Buffy stand for someone saying that to you?! Hell no, she wouldn't. Buffy would do anything to protect her friends. So take a moment to look inside and check in with your inner Buffy. Does your inner Buffy share a quip? Suggest that you go on patrol (just take a walk)? Does she want you to slay the beast who is hurting you? (That's slay with words, not stakes.) Your inner Buffy might make one or all of these suggestions, and then it's up to you to decide what to do. Once you get this feedback, you can consider how you want to further channel Buffy when you respond to that email your boss sent you. The more you channel Buffy, the more you get to experience other parts of yourself. Over time, you may find that the story you had of yourself as a meek person who isn't great with quips or comebacks starts to shift. Maybe you aren't that shy kid in the corner from third grade anymore!

Once you start to notice these thoughts, you're ready for the final boss battle: rewriting part of the story of you. This may take you to some challenging places, including encounters with past and present versions of you—think Link battling Shadow Link[140] or Buffy battling the first Slayer[141] or Storm battling her claustrophobia[142]—as well as encounters with friends, family, and community. In the same way that you can begin to offer compassion to yourself when you think of your depression as an adorable cat (see chapter 3), so too can you begin to change the narrative in all aspects of your life through your interaction with your fandom attachments.

Meaning-Making

The seeds of Therapeutic Fanfiction have been around for a long time, in part because creative storytelling is how human beings cope with tragedy. As we discussed in chapter 1, play and storytelling go hand in hand. And we aren't just talking video games or tabletop gaming here. We're talking about play that stretches back through the ages. If you're a literary nerd or just a fan of the PBS show *Wishbone*, you've probably heard of the Brontë sisters. Emily, Charlotte, and Anne grew up to write some of the greatest works of nineteenth-century English-language literature—*Wuthering Heights*, *Jane Eyre*, and *The Tenant of Wildfell Hall* being the most infamous.[xlviii] But before they could write these novels, they had to survive their hellacious childhood.[143] Born to a tempestuous clergyman, the sisters lost their mother when Anne was only a year old and, in rapid succession, lost both of their elder parentified sisters while all three were still under the age of ten. Together with their brother, Branwell (who would go on to follow in their father's footsteps in more ways than one), the children created a make-believe community called Angria for Branwell's twelve toy soldiers. They wrote novels, newspapers, magazines, and poetry and designed an elaborate history for their make-believe world.[144] If this sounds a lot like play therapy, that's because it is! Or rather it was as close as four children

[xlviii] Yes, we do think that arguments over which sister was the "better" writer or wrote the "most avant-garde" book are utterly unimportant. Not everything needs to be on a hierarchy.

with no in-home therapists could get to play therapy. And as adults, minus Branwell, who never quite got his poetry off the ground, they continued writing themselves into more pleasant environs, writing the independent lives largely denied them by nineteenth-century rural Britain.

What the Brontë sisters were doing—and what we all do when we engage in any kind of fanfic activity—was making meaning. Humans are meaning-making creatures who are constantly in search of it. A human can survive almost any *how* for a *why*.[xlix] Within fandom, meaning abounds. Stories allow fans to make sense of the world around them and to create meaning within both the world of fandom and the world of daily life. One of the great scholars in meaning-making was Viktor Frankl, a psychiatrist who created a style of therapy called logotherapy that focuses solely on man's search for meaning—also the name of his most famous book.[145] His book tells of Frankl's time in Auschwitz and how he came to find meaning under even the most terrible circumstances. One of the pillars of Frankl's work centers around the power of choice. It is perhaps no surprise that Frankl perfected this theory when he was in the camps. While imprisoned, he had lost most of the personal control he once had over his life. Part of how he survived the camps was to retreat back to a place of emotional control. Though he could neither control the events around him nor the actions taken against him nor even the emotions these situations evoked, he could choose *how to respond.* This realization is the foundation of logotherapy, the therapeutic modality he had begun to develop prior to being rounded up and imprisoned but later honed in the camps. This revelation—and his desire to share it with the world—was Frankl's boon or gift from the underworld that he kept safe to bring back from the abyss and share with his community.

Fandom is much more than meets the eye.[l] Our fandom attachments allow us to find meaning in our lives and to make sense of our world and the people around us. Consider all the stories that have helped you through difficult times and the stories that have allowed all of us to bear witness to other people's journeys. *Maus* is a beautiful and heartbreaking example of

---

[xlix] Nietzsche, Frankl, and Campbell all used variations of this idea through the years but gendered the heck out of it. So we've used therapeutic fanfic to improve it.

[l] Like a transformer.

a story of a desperate journey into the camp at Auschwitz and the author's experience interviewing his father to write this work of art.[146] Writing the story of his father's trauma allowed Art Spiegelman to understand his father and, by so doing, make sense of his own experience of transgenerational trauma (more on that in chapter 8). From there, Art was able to decide what family lessons or tools he wanted to keep and what tools he wanted to pass back. By writing *Maus*, Art literally fanficced his own life, similar to the Brontë sisters, and completed his own meaning-making journey.

Fandom fosters meaning and gives fans a language around life's purpose. As you create your vision or shadow boards, you can reflect on the fandom characters who help you make sense of your life when things are hard, those characters who offer a thoughtful answer to all of your questions. For us, one of these characters will always be Special Agent Dale Cooper from *Twin Peaks*.[147] Coop is always ready and waiting to give you a thumb's up, a hearty hug, or a handshake and, of course, his own special wisdom around the importance of daily gifts. So what would Coop suggest as you're going through a hard time? A cup of coffee and a delicious piece of cherry pie? Or maybe it simply sparks meaning to spend time with him virtually in *Twin Peaks* via rewatching seasons 1 and/or 2.[li] Using the language from your fandom can help to make sense of what's happening in your life and can let others know what's going on with you too. Turning to a specific fandom character helps you access and activate the character's role in your life as a guide. Guides or helpers support us in our meaning-making or hero's journey.

Totem

Our fandom attachments can make for great creative opportunities beyond creating traditional and Therapeutic Fanfictions. You might also feel drawn to create fanart or crafts inspired by your heroes. The act of creating in any form allows your brain to experience play and to continue to feel securely connected. It can also be a great opportunity to craft your own personal

[li] Not season 3. If you loved it, we're happy for you. That wasn't the Coop we're attached to.

grounding object or totem. Totems are objects of meaning, history, and magic.[148] Although totems in mainstream media tend to be associated with nonwhite cultures, totems have been a part of the human species since ancient times. However, as white folks, i.e., the ruling class of Western European regions, sought to distance themselves from their more primitive beginnings, they began to speak of their meaningful items as *heirlooms.* The word *totem* began to take on a negative or pejorative meaning. But is a family heirloom china tea set really more advanced than a Ghanaian mask passed down generationally? Obviously not.

For an example of such a totem in fandom, we need look no further than T'Challa, aka Black Panther, and his family ring. This ancestral heirloom reminds T'Challa of his commitment to his family and his loyalty to his community.[149] It grounds him in his role as Black Panther, protector of the realm. N'Jadaka, aka Erik Stevens, aka Killmonger, as a member of the Wakandan royal family,[lii] also has a ring, inherited from his father. This, coupled with the mask he steals from a London Museum, grounds him in his purpose to reconnect with and rejoin the country, Wakanda, and to take back the birthright that he feels was unfairly denied him.

In Therapeutic Fanfiction, you can find an object that evokes meaning for you, or you can make it! Crafting your own totem can be both a centering mindfulness practice and/or a way for you to connect more deeply with the stories and characters that resonate for you. Creating sculpture or a graphic representation of a character with whom you resonate, beading a mala bracelet using fandom inspiration, and/or knitting or crocheting a plush friend are all ways you can create your totem. If you're a Starfleet engineer, perhaps you want to build your own potato clock to remind you to stay grounded like a potato. If binary is more your thing, perhaps you could build a mindfulness app. Or you could use instruments and/or computers to create anything from sweet synth beats to slow guitar jams. Totems can be found or bought from fellow fandom lovers. When we visited Iceland, we took a rock from a *Game of Thrones* filming site, making it our totem.

[lii] At least in the MCU; we acknowledge that this is not canon as far as the comic books are concerned.

Since the ancients, bread has symbolized the energy to continue on one's quest. We hope that as we bid adieu to this chapter, you are taking with you more Therapeutic Fanfiction skills and knowledge. Even though the first few chapters were like a trail of breadcrumbs, we hope that now you have more than a little food for thought.

FANFIC CASE STUDY: *Legend of Zelda,* Goodbye Isn't the End

Having just closed out our trauma work with the Great Deku Tree, we were eagerly anticipating the weekend and our booking at the famous Hyrule Bed and Breakfast run by the always hospitable Mr. and Mr. Darmani of the Goron community. We glance down at our respective watches just as we hear a soft tinkling of bells and a voice reminiscent of Fran Drescher. We look up to see a fluttering of wings and bright sparkling pink light:

"Hello!"

"Is that you, Navi?" We ask. "You haven't been seen since the opener to *Majora's Mask.*"

Navi shakes her wings in a frustrated fashion, filling our tree-house office with a cacophony of bells. "Hey! Listen! This isn't about me. It's about my friend, Link! He's lost and alone and in need of some guidance."

Before we can gently suggest that this seems more like her department, Navi flies up and out the window. With a final jostling of bells, she is gone.

With that, we are on our way again but are once more interrupted, this time by a loud *hup!* We decide that we aren't going to be on time for the bed and breakfast and send a quick apology text. Within moments, a small green-clad figure of questionable age *hups* into our treeway.

"Hi! I'm Link! I can talk now!" While he can now talk, he is still new at it.

"Hello, Link. A friend of yours was just here and seemed worried about you. Would you like to come in?"

Link looks up into our faces with tears in his eyes. "I have friends? . . . I don't remember them. . . . I'm not sure if I remember who I am." He wanders over to a soft chair that looks vaguely like moss. "May I sit?"

"Please." We motion for him to sit and offer him some tea, which he happily accepts. "So, Link, tell us more about what's going on, as much as you can remember."

Link takes a deep breath. "Well, a while ago I woke up in a big cavern with all these glowing blue lights. And I heard this strange ethereal voice, and then I felt annoyed, then excited, then annoyed again. I found my big blue iPhone and set off out of the cavern, where I was immediately attacked by large orange monsters. I don't know how, but I remembered how to fight and vanquished them using a branch I foraged for in some bushes next to the cavern—which might actually have been a temple?" He pauses to take a sip of tea. "This is really good. What did you make it with?

"It's oolong. It comes in a packet."

"Wow, I think I have to make all my food from scratch."

"That sounds really hard. Both the food thing and all of the other stuff, too. It sounds like for all intents and purposes you've been fighting for as long as you can remember. That would be very hard. How can we best support you through this, Link?"

Link furrows his brow. "I . . . I'm not sure if I know what you're asking. All of my memories are jumbled around. The more I try to make sense of them, the more confused I get." Link pauses to study the oolong sloshing around his cup. "This might sound weird but . . . I think I've been a bunch of Links in a lot of different places. Some of those places were definitely Hyrule. But some of them definitely were not."

We look at him with compassionate faces. "That doesn't sound weird at all, Link. Actually, all of us are many people all at once." Link looks a bit confused. "Does *that* sound weird?"

"Hmm, *maybe*. But maybe it also makes sense. Can you explain it more?"

"You bet. So there's this idea in therapy that our minds aren't unitary, meaning that they aren't just one thing, but are in fact many things. We have lots of different parts of ourselves. Some parts want different things than others, but they all want what's best for the person."

"But what if I was different Links in different times? Or in different places? I think I was. I have memories of being much smaller than I am now, and I helped a princess and played an instrument kind of like a flute. But it wasn't a flute. And then I think I was bigger but still playing the not-flute. I met all kinds of beings: Gorons, Kokiri, Zoras. But then it gets jumbled again because the next thing I know I'm small again and I'm sad and my best friend is gone. And I'm in this weird city whose name seems like 'Time' but isn't. And then there's a Twilight place where I'm bigger again but also sometimes a wolf. The worst part is, I don't remember my friends. And I don't know what I'm supposed to be doing here. In all those other times and places, I get the feeling I had a purpose. But I can't remember that either!" Link shakes his mug in frustration, scattering oolong onto the woven mat that doubles as a carpet.

"Wow. That's a lot. No wonder you feel confused and frustrated. It sounds like there are lots of different memories, or parts, that are trying to get your attention. Could we pause for a moment and just take a breath?"

Link looks down at the mat. He says softly, "I'm sorry about your carpet."

"You know what? We wanted to get a new one anyway."

Link looks up and smiles: "Really? So by spilling the tea, I kind of helped you, then?"

"You did! It seems like helping is important to all the iterations of you."

Link takes a deep breath and stares out the window.

We wait for a few moments and then offer: "You can exhale now."

"Oh, right!" Slowly, Link breathes in and out. "I think so. Yes. I think helping has always been . . . part of what I do. Does that make sense?"

"It does. And it also explains why these memories are so loud for you. When our parts are trying to tell us something important, they keep getting louder and louder until we're open to listening to what they have to say. It sounds like your parts are trying to tell you what's important to you and why."

Link chuckles. "I used to know someone who'd get louder and louder . . . to get my attention."

"You did? Do you remember who that was?"

Link closes his eyes. "Navi. I think—her name was Navi. And she meant everything to my destiny. But now she's done." Link opens his eyes as two large tears fall onto his green tunic.

We pause for a moment to allow Link to be with his feelings around this realization. After a few breaths, we offer, "Link, just because someone isn't with us physically doesn't mean that they're gone. What would Navi say if she were here right now?"

"'*HEY! LISTEN!*' in a really screechy voice. She was always telling me things I already knew or was already paying attention to. But, you know, it was nice to have her there to name them."

"She sounds like a really good friend. And even if she can't be with you, she can still help you. You can still call upon her whenever you need her to tell you 'hey, listen' inside your own mind. You are attached to her, and that means that she can be your helper wherever and whenever you need her."

"So . . . she can still help me figure out what I'm doing here?"

"She absolutely can. How about we test that out? Can you take another breath and just turn inward whatever that means to you—maybe close your eyes. And just ask Navi to come forward in your mind. Do you see her?"

Link's eyes are closed so tight that his face is turning red. "*YES!* I do see her! She's a fairy, and she sounds like bells when she moves."

"Great! Now this might sound a little weird, but can you ask the Navi in your mind if she'll talk to us for a little bit?" Link nods. "OK, thank her for being willing to help us out. Now ask if there's something that she wants you to know."

"She says that she wants me to save Hyrule. No. Wait. She's not saying that. That's what all my old memories say. She says . . . she says she wants me to make new friends. She says it might be hard at first but that I can try. I'm better at it than I think." Link bows his head and says softly, "Thanks, Navi."

"That was wonderful, Link. Ask the Navi in your mind if she'd also like to stay with you as you start to make new friends or if she'd like to stay somewhere else where you can find her when you need her."

"She says she wants to stay in the fairy fountain near Goran Pass. She says it's where she was born and it has always been her favorite. I know the way there, so I'll always be able to go back to visit her when I need to. She says I can always visit."

"That's beautiful. Before we say goodbye to her, is there anything else that you'd like to tell the Navi in your mind?"

"I'm sorry for all those times I yelled at you. You were only trying to help. It's just sometimes it's hard to fight boss battles and talk to your friend in a normal speaking voice. That's not an excuse, just context."

"That's very kind of you. How does she respond?"

"She says thank you. She appreciates hearing that."

"Does it feel OK to the both of you to say goodbye for now?"

Link takes a deep, shuddering breath. "I . . . I think so. She'll be happy at the fairy fountain. I wish we'd had more time together. But I probably always would have wanted more time. I love you, Navi."

"That's right. You would always want more time. Take a moment and say goodbye, and take the Navi in your mind to the fairy fountain. We can wait. Just let us know when you're back."

We sit quietly and watch as Link takes several deep breaths, opening and closing his hands. After what feels like both a long and a short time, he opens his eyes and looks around the room.

He blinks. "Hey, I feel better. I actually feel better. How did you do that? Are you a wizard?"

"Nope, we're not wizards, but we have some pretty great wizards in our own minds who help us along the way too."

We look at one another and smile. "Would you like another cup of tea?"

"Yeah," Link says, "I would like that."

FANFIC CASE STUDY QUESTIONS:
Finding Your Inner Fellows

* In the fanfiction case study, who is part of Link's fellowship?
* How does Link's fellowship help him make meaning in his life?
* Who are some of the members of your fellowship?

LEGEND OF ZELDA YOGA:
"Hey Listen!" Follow Your Inner Navi

The purpose of this yoga sequence is to offer grounding while things are difficult. These balancing poses are purposely challenging, so please be kind to yourself if you find that they are difficult, and remember that you can always use a chair or the wall to assist you in your balancing. Imagine that in each pose, Navi appears and shouts, "Hey, listen!"

GREAT DEKU OR TREE POSE

1. Begin with your feet a comfortable distance apart and your arms at your sides.
2. Shift weight onto your left foot, and turn your right knee outward. Feel free to leave your right toes on the floor or have your right heel pressed against your left ankle. As you feel more balanced, you can move your right foot up your left leg as high as is comfortable. (Just avoid your knee joint; your knee will thank you.)
3. Your arms can be wherever you prefer: on your hips, up overhead like a tree, or resting on a chair or the wall for balance. Once you find your balance, try to hold it for three to five full breaths, and then release. Switch sides, and repeat.

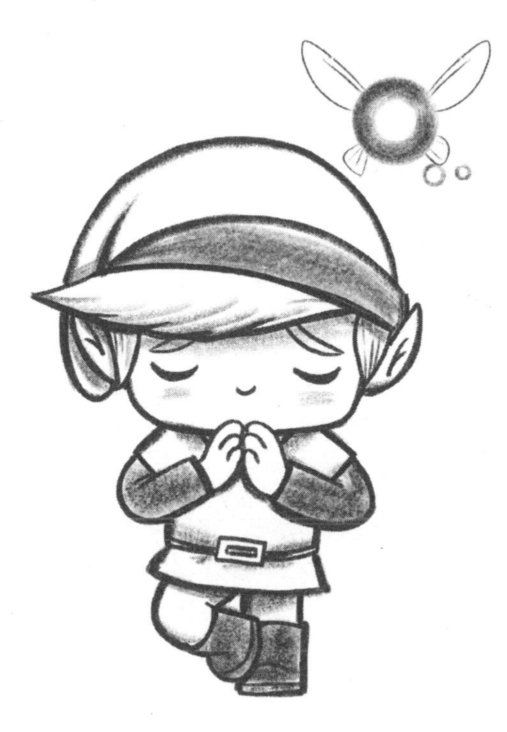

RITO OR EAGLE POSE

1. Begin with your feet a comfortable distance apart and your arms at your sides.
2. Lift arms up overhead, and identify your right hand (hey!).
3. Bring your right arm under your left, giving yourself a hug.

   If you find that you want more stretch and the option is available to you, you can cross your arms at both your elbows and your wrists.
4. Now sit way back in an imaginary chair (we know).

   You're welcome to stay right here; it's a perfectly good spot to be or . . .

   Shift your weight onto your left foot, and bring your right leg up and over the left.

5. Some folks like to cross first and then sit back; some cross just at the ankle. The fun is that you get to make this pose your own!

   Once you find your balance, see if you can hold it for three to five breaths, and then release. Next, try on the other side!

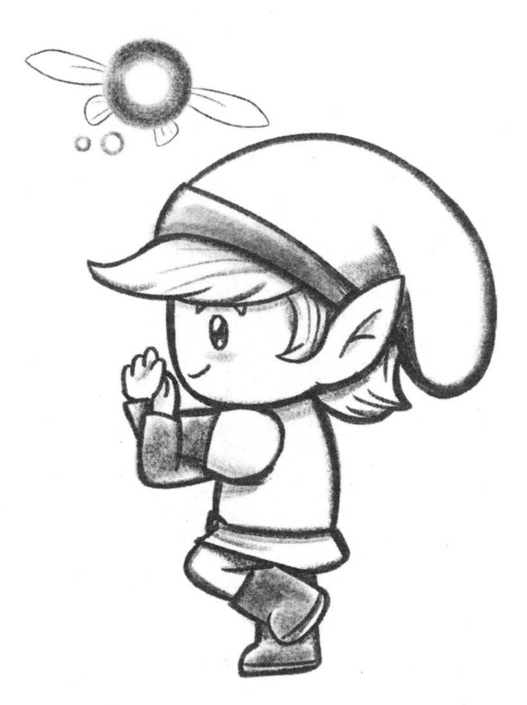

LINK IN FLIGHT OR AIRPLANE POSE

1. Begin with your feet a comfortable distance apart and your arms at your sides.
2. Step your right foot forward.

   Feel free to keep your left toes on the ground, or you can begin to lift that leg as far as is comfortable, but be mindful not to tip your upper body too far forward, or your Link might crash-land.
3. Sweep both arms back behind you.

   Lift your chest like a proud Link.

Balance here for three to five breaths, and feel the Breath of the Wild in your hair. Then release, and repeat while switching sides.

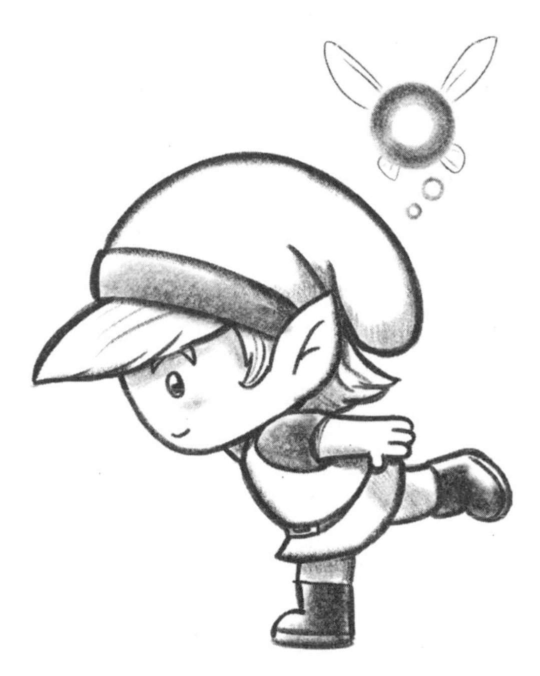

4. Repeat this sequence as many times as sparks joy for you or helps you feel like you indeed have listened to Navi and it's time to get in the game!

When Fandom Betrays Us

Quentin: You think Penny's most prized possession is his Adderall?

Alice: If I had voices all day long telling me to do dark magic and, I don't know, the pills were the one thing that made them stop, they'd be pretty precious.

Quentin: You can always get more pills. They're fungible.

Alice: You're fungible!

—*THE MAGICIANS*, "THE STRANGLED HEART"[150]

Therapeutic Fanfiction can help us rewrite our lives by embracing the narrative powers of myth and stories to help us find the hero within to unlock new power-ups on the greatest of all adventures: the adventure of our lives. By using the tools of the Westworld Construct, externalizing the problem, personification, fandom attachment, and rewriting your story, you're learning how to become the Buffy you seek. Perhaps you're thinking to yourself that all of this sounds great but you've already been using coping skills to deal with your problems and it's been working well . . . enough.[liii] We're sure that's true. We are all skilled at figuring out ways to cope in the short term, but just because these short-term solutions work well . . .

[liii] Shout out to those readers who picked up on this deep cut reference from our podcast.

enough doesn't mean that they're serving you as much as they could be. Perhaps these maladaptive coping skills, or, as we call them, shadow tools, are causing more difficulties for you in the future. Some of the coping skills we turn to that have a shadow aspect include, but are certainly not limited to, drinking, drugging, and hooking up with strange pieces (à la *The LEGO Movie*),[151] and other forms of self-harm in all of its various permutations. Let's pause for a moment and consider what shadow tools you tend to opt for. Take a moment and reflect in your journal or your mind-palace.

Shadow Tools of Dean Winchester

Whereas you might look at this list and label these behaviors "bad," we don't like to moralize any behaviors. In fact, these behaviors serve a purpose, right? They help us take our mind off of the thing at hand, which allows us to move forward, but, unfortunately, they also cause us to feel shame and may also leave behind other scars, both physical and emotional. One of our most beloved maladaptive fandom copers is Dean Winchester of *Supernatural* fame.

Dean has been through a lot over the course of his, well, life. And he never learns how to regulate his emotions, nor how to handle discomfort when external events feel out of control. So Dean figures out that he can cope with his feelings through drinking, eating copious amounts of pie, and hooking up with strange small-town servers. And while those things help him get through the day or the moment, they don't get to the root of his feelings. The feelings are still there even as the waitress heads back to her next shift at the bar. What might happen if Dean actually deals with some of his shit—like, really deals with it? We're not sure he would even know what that looks like. He and brother Sammy have had so very many conversations about their feelings,[liv] but they never truly hear one another. And yes, there are some systemic challenges to them making authentic change in their lives. But if they could work as a team against their common problem instead of fighting one another, they just might be happier and healthier.

[liv] Fifteen seasons' worth of conversations to be exact.

Perhaps you're thinking, *Wait, I know what Sammy and Dean can do!* Yes, they can use all the pain and trauma from losing their mother at a very young age, off-roading on numerous demon hunting trips with dad, and the loss of numerous friends and chosen family[152] duc to, again, monsters, by using the tool of posttraumatic growth. They can grow through their pain and come out the other side stronger, smarter, stealthier.

The path of posttraumatic growth is in some ways laid out before Sam and Dean, calling them to walk forth. However, the brothers are missing some of the systemic criteria that would make posttraumatic growth possible. Recall from chapter 4 that, to grow from a traumatic situation, a person needs supportive community, a clear sense of purpose, that is, a meaning for suffering, and time to reflect on pain. While Dean and Sam clearly have the tool of community and a tome of meaning—symbolized as a literal tome in the series as the hunter's journal—they don't exactly have a lot of time to reflect on their pain. Their core caregivers, biological Papa Winchester and adoptive father Bobby,[lv] differ in some dramatic ways, but they align in their commitment to drinking away feelings. To further complicate matters, Sam and Dean often feel trapped in a hero's journey without end, one that deprives them of the crucial final step of returning to the community to reintegrate both themselves and their hard-won gift. Deprived of this final restorative stage, Sammy and Dean cling to each other and their hunter's journey ever tighter. And as their alienation from the larger nondemon outside world increases, so too does their use of shadow tools.

So what are some examples of coping skills that represent the light? Well, some options in times of crisis would be to reach out to your friends or chosen family. When Dean's having a hard time, instead of hooking up with waitstaff, he could call his very, *very* good friend and life partner Castiel[lvi] and talk about how he's feeling. The dude's an angel; he gets it. Or Dean could try journaling. He already has a pretty sweet hunter's journal, but what if, in addition to listing all the big bads and the ways to dust

---

[lv] RIP

[lvi] Yes, we ship Destiel. If you don't, we salute and respect your choices, while asking that you prepare for more Destiel references. Because, in the words of Sweet Dee Reynolds, "it's gonna happen."

them, he also reflects on the events of the hunt and the feelings that came up for him? We recommend keeping a hunter's journal. We're all fighting demons on the regular—whether it's a literal monster under the bed or a metaphorical monster in upper management. It helps to keep a record of events, the tools that helped us defeat the demon, and our emotional reactions to the struggle. Other options for your hunter's toolkit include getting some exercise, like Sammy who regularly goes for a jog even when he isn't hunting a Rugaru. Dean definitely does not jog, but if he were to check out some other wellness activities, he might find that he's super into cycling, or weightlifting, or Zumba. He just won't know until he tries. Also, we'd like to pitch the idea of classic rock Zumba, because "Carry on Wayward Son" would just kick ass with a box step move.

Stress Mountain

Hopefully, a pattern is starting to emerge. We aren't just talking about coping when things are bad; we're talking about setting up a lifestyle wherein we are taking care of ourselves regularly so that our distress tolerance is raised and our likelihood of spawning gremlins or accidentally inviting in the Depressogorgon is lowered. We don't all start from the same place with regard to our distress tolerance. Stress Mountain is a metaphor we often use with clients to help them visualize the ways that systems impact our stress levels. Factors like socioeconomic status, race, gender, ethnicity, as well as our personal history determine where we start on Stress Mountain, which tells us how much room we have to roam.

Let's look at Stress Mountain:

A. This is absolute zero, the bottom of the mountain, where stress is nonexistent. Literally nobody lives here. No, not even monks in a cave. They need to worry about what the humidity might do to their singing bowls. They still have stress.

B. This is Sharknado Peak, also called Shitstorm Peak or Ganon Peak (or insert-your-fandom-here Peak), where stress has become so high so as to become unmanageable. Here, you have much lowered distress tolerance, and you're likely to yell at your partner for loading the dishwasher "wrong."

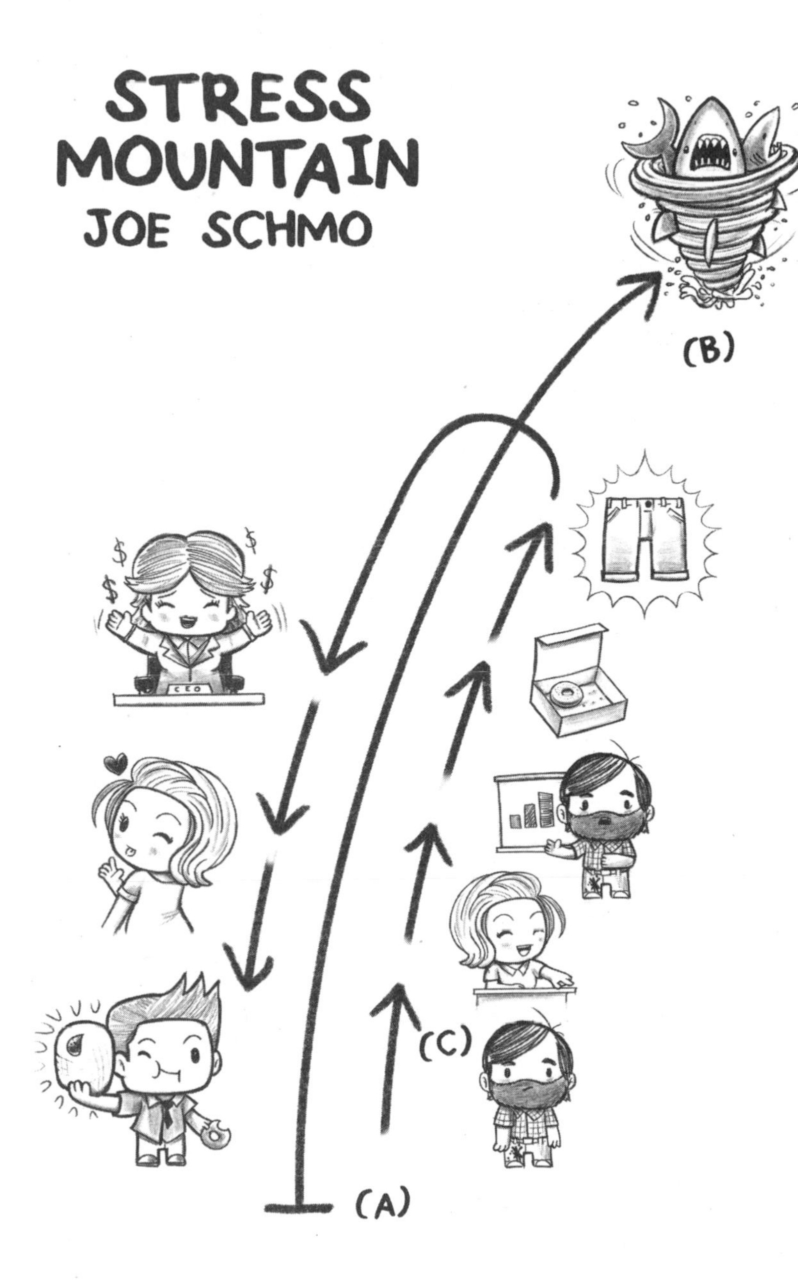

C. Let's look at an example of a regular Joe, Joe Schmo. He's an upper-middle-class cisgender, heterosexual white man with two loving parents who have been married for forty years, and he's managed to have a lifetime of secure attachments to other human beings. Yet even Joe can have a rough day that has him traveling up Stress Mountain.

Imagine that on this day, as Joe is driving to work enjoying his caramel macchiato and rocking out to Journey, he accidentally spills it all over his khakis. Dangit! It's too late to turn around and go home, so he has to go into work with his coffee-khakis. And he moves up the mountain. He encounters the nice woman at the front desk, and she giggles about his misadventure. He moves further up. Then he remembers the big presentation he has to give today, and he moves further up the mountain. But, thankfully, he remembers that today is donut day and goes to the breakroom for his jelly-filled only to find the box jelly-less. He moves up again. But without any actual effort, his day starts to course-correct. He gets a call from the laundry service he uses saying that his week's laundry is done and he can get fresh khakis at lunch. And he moves down the mountain. Then he rocks his presentation; with his boss happy, he moves down. Then he sees the pretty woman at the front desk who smiles at him, and he moves down. And finally, but perhaps most importantly, his work-bro comes to see him and surprises him with a jelly-filled donut. They weren't gone; his work-bro just knew they are his favorite and saved one for him. See, Joe moved way up the mountain but was able to course-correct before he got anywhere near his Sharknado Peak.

But look what happens if your life circumstances have you starting much further up the mountain:

D. Here you see our beloved bowlegged Dean Winchester starting his day about two arrows from a shark. By the time Dean finishes a demon hunt, he's almost out of room, so when Sammy wants to have a brotherly moment, Dean has been half devoured by sharks. Unlike Joe Schmo, Dean can't just naturally course-correct. Dean has already reached shark food; thus, he needs to do a lot of conscious self-care to start to move back down the mountain. But he only manages to move himself about the same distance each day, which means it's Tuesday and tomorrow is Tuesday and every day is Tuesday.[lvii] If Dean were

[lvii] *Supernatural*, Season 3, episode 11, "Mystery Spot."

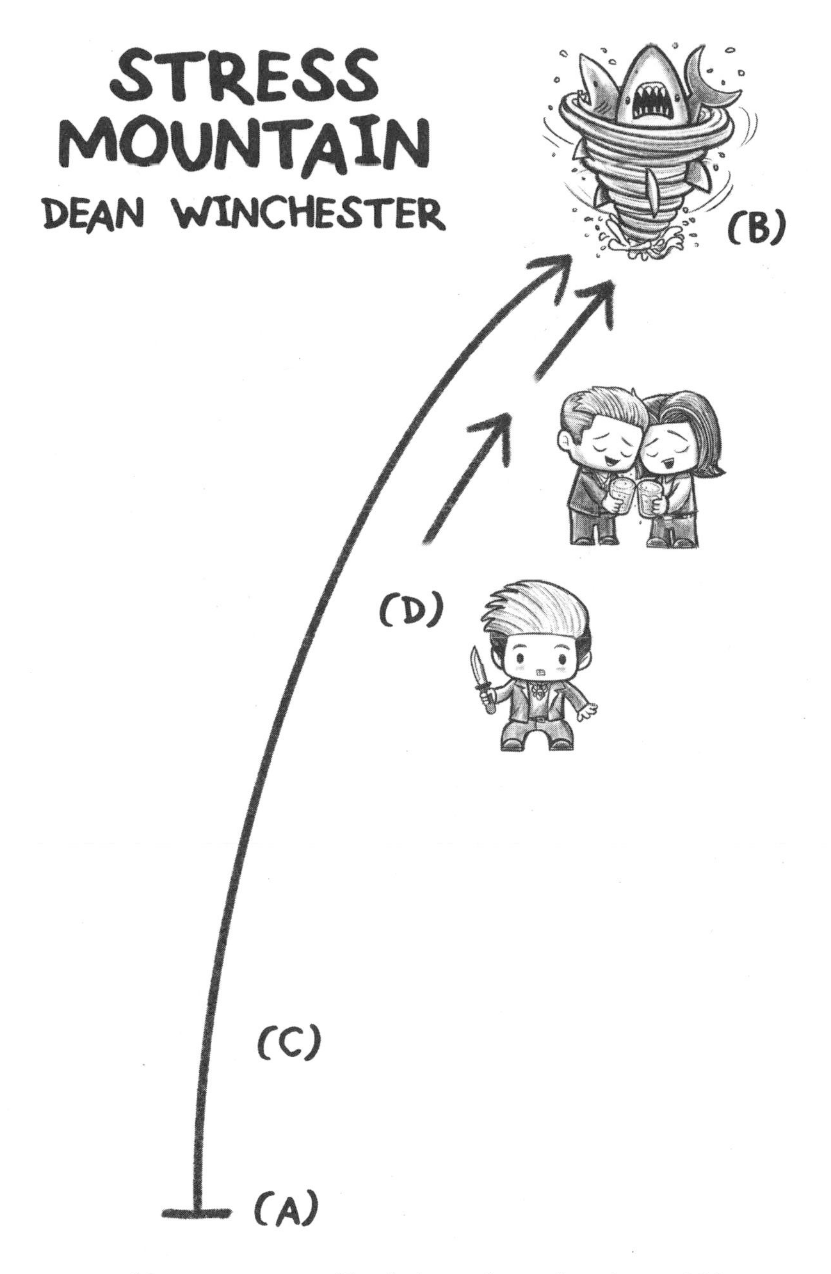

able to put some of his light tools in place, he could begin to move down the mountain so that when stress arises, he has more room to roam. Not only is taking care of yourself a radical, political act, but it is also a vital part of your own survival and thrival.

The Shadow Side of Fandom Attachment

One of the great ways that we can take care of ourselves is through our relationship with stories, as you, reader, are well aware. But even these fandom attachments can have a shadow side to them. It is possible to become so invested in fandom attachments that we lose some balance in our lives, meaning that we let our IRL attachments dwindle. It's important to have both. And it's also important to remember that fandom attachments, while so helpful and healing, are one-sided.[153] They can only support us inasmuch as we allow them to support us.[154] Their help is limited.

Remember all the way back to chapter 1 when we talked about the difference between a character and their actor? Here we build on that idea. Something that can happen for folks when they get the opportunity to meet their fandom favorites is that they overshare. They don't mean to cause harm; in fact, they truly want to thank the performer for helping them through a hard time. When you go to a comic convention where you've spent possibly thousands of dollars to have only moments with the object of your fandom attachments, you might scream, "I love you!" or share with the celebrity the number of times the celebrity has helped you through personal challenges. This disclosure is a bid to attach and to set yourself apart from the crowd of others who are shouting their praise.

But there's some confusion around boundaries (more on that in chapter 7). You, the fan, don't know the actor, even though you know the character. At their core, boundaries are about consent: what one is consenting to share and what others are consenting to hear. In the case of celebrity appearances at conventions, many fans make statements that the celebrity does not consent to hearing. Although public figures open themselves up to certain discourse, celebrities have not consented to verbal, emotional, or physical intimacy.

Our fandom attachments are very real, and the place that characters hold in our communities exists. The key point to remember is that a celebrity is the placeholder or representation of this emotional relationship. Though social media has expanded the ability to engage with the representatives of these characters, this engagement creates a false sense of closeness to the person. Celebrities or influencers may use this space to foster the sense of an IRL connection to increase their own popularity, but this closeness is an illusion that simply makes use of the fandom attachment that you have created with the imagined version of them that lives in your own headcanon.

Both an IRL friend and a fandom attachment friend can offer support and loving kindness. Part of what makes meditation, visualization, and Therapeutic Fanfiction so powerful is that our emotions don't distinguish between what we imagine to be real and what we are experiencing in real time. So when we imagine General Leia Organa[155] or Buffy Summers rallying us to face the day with an inspiring speech and loving gaze, our emotions react just as they would if Leia really was in our bedroom telling us that we truly can face Pam in accounting.

The difference in our experience has to do with intensity—or quantity—of these emotions, as well as control. If General Organa were actually in your bedroom, you would still feel what you feel when you imagine her, but you would feel it more intensely.[lviii] You might also find an emotion to be present that isn't nearly so intense (or perhaps isn't there at all) when you were just imagining her: fear, because, OMG, General Organa is literally in your bedroom and what do you even say to her? Fandom attachment gives you control over the imagined scenario while giving you the emotional payoff of Leia's guidance without risking becoming overwhelmed by feelings and/or panic.

As powerful as our fandom attachments and imagined scenarios are, they are not a replacement for IRL attachment. The avatars Leia, Buffy, and Sam Winchester cannot engage in real-time feedback and reciprocal communication, both of which are key components of a corrective emotional experience. In other words, our imagination is a beautiful and incomparable place, and we also need to get actual feedback from other human beings to heal. In this case, as in many others, the situation calls for *both/and* not *either/or*.

[lviii] It might be helpful to think of it in terms of math. When you imagine General Organa, you will feel five units of joy, but were she actually in your bedroom you would feel fifty units of joy.

Corrective Emotional Experiences

A *corrective emotional experience* is often a part of posttraumatic growth.[156] It's an opportunity to mitigate your use of, or need for, shadow tools and to reexperience yourself as a worthy human being through compassionate interaction with a fellow human. If this sounds complicated, don't worry. The act of reading this book involves you taking part in a potentially corrective emotional experience. So take a deep breath, and let's try this out.

Below, you'll find a short list of fandom characters who eventually find ways to heal through restorative connection with other living beings. We're being as generic as possible here because humans aren't the only people with whom you can engage in healing connection. Have you ever had a dog? Or loved a cat? Whispered sweet nothings to your grove of indoor plants (they provide you oxygen; it's reciprocal)? Then you get it.

As you read through this short list, we invite you to pause at least once per paragraph and practice noticing your feelings. If you notice yourself having a feeling or five, try naming what they are. You might notice sadness, shame, fear, and/or anger. As you continue reading, you might notice these feelings either shifting or being joined by other feelings: hope, reassurance, humor, and/or joy. This confluence of feelings is part of what we're talking about with the phrase *corrective emotional experience.*

Perhaps the character Dean Winchester best resonates with your own struggle with shadow tools. But maybe you've never watched *Supernatural* and aren't keen to start.[lix] If you're a comic book fan, Old Man Logan, aka *X-Men*'s Wolverine, is a great example of a character who has struggled and suffered with the idea that he is fundamentally flawed and unworthy of love and affection.[157] Like Dean, Logan often turns to alcohol to numb his pain and detach from "bad memories." Whether you're a fan of the Netflix series or a die-hard for the Brian Michael Bendis comic books, Jessica Jones is another great example of a hero who struggles with shame, guilt, and superpowers.[158] Like Logan and Dean, Jessica often turns to her old friend whiskey to help numb the pain and disconnect from painful feelings.[159]

[lix] We get it; at fifteen seasons with twenty-three or twenty-four episodes per season, it's a real time commitment.

The irony here is that the more you drink, the more you feel and the more you feel, the more you drink. Penny of *The Magicians* uses pain pills and sex to cope with the very real problem of hearing other people's thoughts and feelings all the damn time.[160] This is a great example of using a shadow tool to cope with a serious problem. In the short term, both sex and pain medications help Penny to tune out the trauma of the world and tune into whatever is in front of him, be it a magical tome or a magic crazed sociopath known as the Beast. If your fandom takes a more literary bent, Emily Brontë's Heathcliff might come to mind as a heroic antihero whose orphan status marks him as too lowly to pursue his one true love, Cathy.[161] So instead he walks the moors, bottle in hand, raging at the world and, sometimes, at Cathy herself.

For each of these characters, healing takes time and comes in fits and starts. Not all of them are able to sustain and increase the healing they experience through their respective corrective emotional experiences. Logan benefits from the positive connection he fosters with father figure Charles Xavier and a series of adopted children: Kitty Pryde, Jubilee, and X-23. Jessica Jones begins to heal when she starts to open up and trust her friend Carol Danvers in the comics or Trish in the Netflix series. Penny has a more complicated emotional journey in both iterations of himself: timeline 23 Penny and timeline 40 Penny. And Heathcliff, well, his status as a foundling and questionable ethnic and racial background coupled with his doomed love of Cathy are pretty much the kiss of death. He gets some emotionally corrective moments but not enough to build on, as his external surroundings thwart him at every turn. Being on the wrong side of privilege is brutal.

For our money, one of the best examples of the healing powers of IRL connection happens to *Mass Effect*'s Mordin. Introduced in *Mass Effect 2*, Mordin is an alien scientist, a Salarian scientist to be exact, onboard Commander Shepard's ship, the *Normandy*, and his claim to fame is creating a genetic virus that decimated an alien species called the Krogan.[162] Mordin's shadow tool of choice is work; he spends a lot of *Mass Effect 2* working really hard to avoid too much interpersonal connection.[lx] In *Mass Effect 3*,

---

[lx] He isn't even a romance option! Le sigh.

Mordin and Commander Shepard have the opportunity to cure the genetic virus that Mordin created and to help the Krogans heal. Players selecting this path get to experience Mordin coming alive to himself. He sings, he makes jokes, and he even openly befriends his Krogan patient, Eve. If you haven't played *Mass Effect 3*, we couldn't recommend it more, and we don't want to spoil it or Mordin's ending.[163] Suffice it to say, Mordin has the chance to become the healing force he always wanted to be. In his own words, "It had to be me. Someone else would have gotten it wrong."

If you haven't noticed at least one feeling yet, that might mean that the fandom characters described above don't particularly resonate for you, and that is understandable! Use some Therapeutic Fanfiction skills to sub characters that hit you right in the feels.

Now you're ready for the final step. For the process of the corrective emotional experience to complete, you'll need to take the next step and share these feelings with another creature that you trust. If that feels overwhelming, that is also totally normal! As anyone who resonates with Dean Winchester might tell you, expressing feelings initially seems like a lot less fun than five bottles of beer and a whole pie. But here's the thing: though pie and beer can feel great in the moment, they eventually lead to a sugar crash and bloat. We're not telling you not to eat pie. But we are encouraging you to think about what coping strategies might serve you best in both the long and short term. Sometimes, the answer might be pie and two beers. And sometimes, it might be asking your best baby bro to go get some pie with you and—gulp!—talk about those eggshells you've been walking on since Sammy's lady friend left the bunker.

FANFIC CASE STUDY: *Supernatural*, Saving Memories, Hunting Shame—the Family Legacy

After a yearlong stint as in-home therapists in the gaming universe of Hyrule, we decide to spend some time in environs that bring back memories of our midwestern youth: the windswept plains of Lawrence, Kansas, where stories go to end... or is it begin? At any rate, we just finished setting up our office when we hear the waiting room door open and shut, and then open and shut again. Distant sounds of swearing and grumbling could be heard.

We walk the few steps out to the entryway to find a compact yet beautiful man scanning the waiting room uneasily as he shifts from one booted foot to the next, bowleggedly making his way back toward the front door. "Can we help you?"

"Son of a bitch! Sorry, I mean, yeah, I'm, uh, I'm looking for the Jefferson Starships? I mean, Starship doctors? Or Starship therapists? Ugh, I'm gonna kill Sammy. Listen, your name is weird, but my specialty is weird, so why the hell not..." He clears his throat and reaches for the flask clearly outlined in his left breast pocket but then thinks better of it. "Are you the... spaceship guys, er, ladies?" He makes an attempt at a smile—and possibly a wink? We decide to definitely take it personally.

"Why don't you come in and tell us what's going on... uh..."

"Dean. Dean Winchester. Monster hunter, Aquarius, beach walker, lover of frisky women. And men."

"Good to meet you, Dean." Once we settle into our office, Dean's demeanor changes, and he seems markedly on edge. No longer thinking about leaving, he is in a heightened state of vigilance. We offer him some tea. He makes a face that we take for a no and move on. "Could you tell us a bit about what brought you here today? We gather it wasn't entirely your choice. You mentioned a Sammy?"

"My kid brother, though he's big as a moose. He said I need to 'feel my feelings' and, I dunno, maybe I do? My childhood was real messed up, and my adulthood, well, it ain't any better."

"That sounds hard, Dean. How do you deal with things being so difficult?"

"You just keep swinging. It's the only way. I'll go down swinging."

We exchange glances. "It sounds like you've been fighting all your life. When you aren't fighting, Dean, what do you do? Who is important to you?"

He shifts uncomfortably in his chair, and, already almost on the very edge, he nearly falls. He steadies himself in a manner that plays to a desire for utter coolness.

"My family is most important to me. Family is all I've got: Sammy, Cass, and Jack. I lost my mom when I was a kid, although I got her back for a while . . . long story. My dad was an ass, but I loved him, man how I looked up to him . . ." Dean pauses as a single tear runs down his cheek. "Got to see him one last time too. A big, dysfunctional family dinner." We pause and allow Dean to sit with his feelings. "So, can you fix me? Or am I too far gone?"

We smile kindly at him. "Fixing isn't what we do, Dean. We don't believe in broken. You've had so much loss in your life. You didn't have people to show you how to cope with it all. People think that somehow we all just inherently know how to take care of ourselves, but that isn't true. We learn how to do it, and, unfortunately, you were alone a lot."

Dean continues to cry softly. "I had Bobby. Bobby was there."

"Tell us about Bobby."

"Bobby was the absolute best. Dad would leave us with him when we were kids, and he would take me out to just play ball. He was a hunter, too, but we weren't always hunting. But we definitely didn't talk feelings. Bobby drank. He lost his wife, and I know there was something about his folks, but he never told us. I guess all I've ever known how to do is get through the day with a bottle, a girl—no offense—and some Zeppelin."

"Well, we can't argue with Zeppelin."

Dean looks up, quickly wiping away his tears. "Yeah? You two fans?" We nod. "I didn't know they played Zeppelin on the Jefferson Starship."

We chuckle and offer, "Learned all kinds of things in therapy school."

"Yeah, I'll bet. I always thought Sammy should have gone in for that. He used to think he wanted to be a lawyer, but I never saw him that way.

Sammy wasn't an arguer, not really. He sure likes talking about feelings. Opening up. Never had an experience he didn't want to talk about."

"What's that like for you, Dean?"

"For me? It's fuckin' weird and not the Djinn kinda wierd. Djinns, vampires—gimme a Rugaru, and I'm good for the day. But, honestly, I don't know what feelings are even for. What good do they do you? They just make you freeze up when you gotta move, blink when you gotta stay focused. My first fight—well, my first hunt—I nearly got my dad killed because I was so busy feeling I couldn't even hold the crossbow straight."

"How old were you, Dean?"

"That doesn't matter. A hunter always has to be ready."

We hold the silence for a few breaths and then:

"I was eight," he says.

"You were eight."

"Yeah, but I still shouldn't've froze up. That was stupid."

"Dean, have you interacted with an eight-year-old recently?"

Dean thinks for a moment. "Yeah, guess I saved one not too long ago, why?"

"How would you describe that eight-year-old?"

"Uh, I dunno, some stupid kid . . . wait . . . we're all just stupid fucking kids, aren't we? It wasn't fair what the old man asked me to do."

"No, Dean, it wasn't fair. Your dad experienced a terrible loss, and he couldn't take care of himself. You stepped up and did things that were way out of the scope of a little kid. Now the challenge is learning how to be your own parent. How to be the dad you didn't get. Not for Sammy, not for Jack. Just for you."

Dean's voice catches in his throat: "Wha—what about me?"

"You're important, too, Dean."

"I guess. . . . But what am I supposed to do with these feelings? You seriously do not expect me the next time I encounter a Rugaru to just *feel* at him do you?"

"Well, not exactly, no. But you might try feeling *afterward*."

"What would that even look like?" Dean reaches into his pocket and fidgets with the flask.

"Well, this might sound strange, but have you ever . . . journaled?"

Dean scoffs, "You kidding me? All the time. How else am I going to keep track of all the monsters we hunt and how to kill them? Jesus! I'm smart, but I'm not encyclopedia smart. I write it down so I can, you know, reference it later."

"OK, great! So you're already an experienced journaler. How about adding just a bit to that. What if in addition to adding info about the beasts, you also talked about what it was like for you to hunt, about how you felt and how this particular time impacted you and your family?"

"That sounds weird."

"And monster hunting isn't?"

"Touché, Jefferson Starship, touché. OK, so I write down my feelings and then what?"

"Well, first you can bring those thoughts and feelings in here and share them with us. And then we'll look at the ways that you deal with difficult feelings, and you can decide whether or not those coping skills are serving you or harming you. And you might decide to change some behavior. And then at some point maybe you share what's going on with Sammy or Cass or Jack. But that's all down the road. For now, just write down the feelings without judging them or yourself." Dean just stares for a moment.

"This may be the hardest thing I've ever done."

We nod. "It is. But if it wasn't hard, it wouldn't be important."

FANFIC CASE STUDY QUESTIONS:
Finding Coping Strategies, Making Lists, Moving Forward

* Using what you've learned in the chapter, list some self-care practices and habits that Dean could engage in both in the moment and on a daily basis instead of the tried-and-true sex, booze, quips, and pie.

* Now, list some self-care strategies that might be helpful on a regular basis for Dean and for yourself.
* What are some ways that you could incorporate these self-care practices into your daily life?
* What are some self-care strategies that might prove especially helpful during times of crisis or stress?

MEDITATION FOR GROUNDING:

"Sitting in the Impala," a Meditation on Finding the Power of Coming Home to Oneself

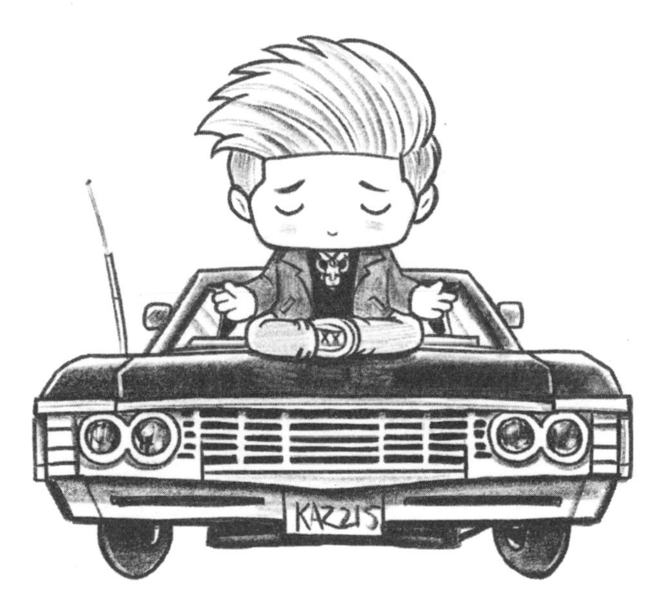

Sam and Dean Winchester's beloved 1967 black Chevrolet Impala feels like home. When they are in the car, they experience a feeling of safety, even when life feels very dangerous. The Impala is deeply meaningful to the brothers, and it is truly a *grounding object,* a physical reminder of a mental state. This meditation hopes to create the same feeling of connection no matter what your grounding object might be.

While you can meditate in any position, it might be most helpful (particularly if meditating is new for you) to start with your feet flat on the floor, arms at your sides or in your lap (or holding this book if paper books are your jam). You might try softening the edges of your eyelids. Once you've shifted into a more physically relaxed position, we invite you to tune into your breathing. You might try three to five deep breaths, in through your nose and out through the mouth. If you're like us, you might not be able to breathe through your nose right now because #sinusstruggles, and that's all right. Rather than breathing like you're being chased by a yellow-eyed demon, we invite you to breathe like you're chilling out and listening to some classic rock.

Now, imagine yourself in the Chevy Impala, bringing your attention to the feeling of your feet on the floor of the car. You might notice the feeling of your feet against your socks and then the feeling of your feet in heavy durable boots, excellent for out-running demons. For now, imagine that there are no demons who need vanquishing. There are no fellow humans who need saving. There is only you, the Impala, and the lull of the wind as it blows through the grass.

Take a deep breath in . . . and a deep breath out. We invite you to tune into your sense of sound. Perhaps you imagine the purr of the engine as it carries you to parts unknown. Perhaps your Impala is parked on the side of the road overlooking a river and you notice the thrushing sound of steady waves against the riverbank. Whatever you hear, breathe into it. Allow the muscles in your feet and legs to relax.

Take a deep breath in . . . and a deep breath out. As you shift your attention to another of your five senses, we invite you to notice the smells of the interior. Perhaps you notice the calming scent of musk and leather. Perhaps you detect a hint of wet grass after rain. Whatever smells you notice, allow them to be just as they are. There is no call to action here.

Allow your attention to shift up from your legs to your stomach or torso, drawing the rooted energy of the Impala up through your feet, through your legs, and into your solar plexus. Notice the feeling of your back against the seat of the Impala. Allow yourself to lay back into the cushions supporting your back, neck, and spine. Take a deep breath in . . . and a deep breath out.

You may notice that you have been breathing deeply for a while now. Slowly begin to refocus the gaze of your mind on the open road. Perhaps you see a sunrise, the light of the sun reaching out across gray-blue skies. Perhaps the sun is setting, withdrawing into the dim of twilight. Whatever you see, let it be pleasing and comforting. You are safe, you are held, and you are protected within the Impala.

Before you put the key in the ignition, before you switch the radio dial over to the classic rock station, shift your attention inward, and set an intention for this next journey. Notice any fears or worries that come up for you. Notice any hopes or future plans. Take a deep breath in. Hold the intention clearly in your mind's eye. And as you breathe out, release the intention out into the multiverse. When you are ready, turn the key, and head back out onto the road.

You are ready for another day on your hunter's journey.

Talk Nerdy to Me

I think... that if you love someone, you don't get to choose how they love you back.

—HOA IN *THE STONE SKY, THE BROKEN EARTH: BOOK THREE*[164]

For those who ship Margo and Eliot, from the delightful[lxi] Syfy show *The Magicians,*[165] one of the issues that causes them the most difficulty in their polyamorous relationship is emotional honesty or emotional vulnerability. *The Magicians* explores the magic side of our world by following a group of magical graduate school students through their adventures and sexual escapades.[lxii] Something that *The Magicians* does well is look at poly relationships without judgment. It is possible to have multiple ethically nonmonogamous relationships with others. We won't dive into poly relationships explicitly in this chapter but we will discuss romantic relationships generally, which you can feel free to translate into whatever type of relationships you choose.

This chapter will, amongst other topics, explore ways to honestly commit to another human in a romantic context as well as the ways our earliest intimate relationships in our family of origin or first intimate social group

---

[lxi] And very sweary

[lxii] It's like NC-17 Hogwarts.

impact the ways we both seek out and build romantic connection. It might be helpful to think of the romantic relationship that exists between two or more people as a LEGO bridge and the LEGO blocks as the rules, roles, and boundaries used to build this relationship bridge. The more mindful attention you are able to bring to building this bridge, the stronger your romantic relationship will be. It's important to look back to the rules, roles, and boundaries of your youth to understand how you learned the ones you hold today; using the LEGO analogy, there's a reason that you choose the blocks you did.

Rules

If it's comfortable for you to do so, think back to your family of origin—the folks you grew up with. Now think of what the rules were in your home. We imagine that you're coming up with some concrete things, like, stay out of direct sunlight and don't eat after midnight—or maybe that was only in Gizmo's family of origin. But in addition to those concrete rules, think a bit more about what were the unspoken rules, such as not discussing family business outside the home or needing to keep Uncle Moishe from driving after Passover Seder because he really overdoes it on the Manischewitz.[166] Can you think of any such rules from your own family? We bet you can. As you consider these rules, we invite you to make notes if that's helpful and to do so without placing judgment on those rules or yourself for having followed them. Every family has rules—both spoken and unspoken—and rarely do the Baby Yodas of these families have much say in what these rules will be or how they will be implemented. Sometimes when we revisit these rules as adults it can be hard to think about the memories that arise. If big feelings are coming up for you right now, we invite you to pause. You might need to take a break from reading to journal, spend time with a friend (IRL or fandom), and maybe talk to your own therapist or mentor.

If you feel able to continue but notice some uncomfortable memories, we invite you to recall the loving kindness meditation from earlier in chapter 4. Remember, loving kindness encompasses the idea of self-compassion or the practice of extending kindness and understanding to one's self. Let's revisit our Baby Yoda example. Baby Yoda, of *The Mandalorian*[167] and internet-meme fame, did not have control over the adults attempting to guard, protect, or control them. In fact, when Mando first finds them, Baby Yoda is surrounded by a camp of assassins whose rules seem to be that Baby Yoda stays hidden pretty much at all times in their Death Star bassinet,[lxiii] never plays with other children, and must minimize their curiosity. Clearly, these rules are not in Baby Yoda's best interest, not the least of which because these rules neither acknowledge Baby Yoda's agency nor facilitate Baby Yoda's growth and development. Perhaps, when Baby Yoda grows up, they will reflect back on this early time with sadness. Such a feeling would be totally understandable. However, were grown Baby Yoda to move from sadness to regret, this could easily lead to self-blame, because regret is a feeling that implies responsibility. But Baby Yoda was not empowered to make or change the rules governing their childhood "family" system. Baby Yoda was at the mercy of their "caregivers."

If you are struggling with self-compassion, it may help to try extending self-compassion to a younger or childhood version of you. Remember, younger you had a younger brain. As adults we tend to think back to our younger selves and give them adult thoughts and feelings, but this isn't fair. We had a younger, i.e., less fully developed, brain with younger thoughts and feelings. This is important to remember, especially around feelings of *I should've known better* or *Why did I do that?!* If even picturing a younger version of you feels too hard, use Baby Yoda as a stand-in for your inner child. You might even want to close your eyes and picture Baby Yoda with their cute long ears and inquisitive eyes. Who could be mad at such a lovable creature? Not us and probably not you.

Now that you've started to shine a light on the rules you inherited from your family of origin, we invite you to reflect on the rules that you hold in romantic relationships. Notice which rules mimic those from your family of origin and which differ. Ask yourself, *What rule blocks do I want to keep and what blocks do I want to metaphorically pass back to the family that raised me?*

[lxiii] Although we recognize that this Death Star bassinet is not canon, it is very much a part of our headcanon and we offer it to you to add to your headcanon if you so choose. Even if you don't, you must admit that Baby Yoda's floating bassinet looks a lot like a Death Star.

Roles

Often, the roles we take on in our romantic relationships are informed by the roles we either had or observed in our family of origin.[168] What are some of the roles that you recall from your family of origin? Some concrete answers might come to mind like "mother," "father," and "Uncle Moishe." But there are subtler spoken or unspoken roles. When you think of the concrete answers "child" and "sibling," consider what you did in the family. Were you the one who tried to make everybody laugh when things were rough? Did you try to do super well in school—and everywhere, really—because you didn't want your family to have one more thing to worry about? Or did you maybe get in a lot of trouble, drinking, using drugs, and basically feeling terrible about it? All of those ways that you might have shown up (and infinite others) comprise your role in the family. Some of the most common roles we see in our practice are the parentified child,[169] parent as victim, the spousified child,[170] parent as best friend, the scapegoat,[171] the golden child, and the problem child. You may notice that we are speaking more about children than about parents. That is because we have all been children, but we have not all been parents.

The role of the parentified child is one of the most common that we hear about in our practice. A child becomes parentified when they are asked to do more than is developmentally appropriate for them to handle.[172] In this case they're playing the role of parent to their own caregivers and siblings. Recall Dean Winchester's fanfic case study: Dean talks about his father asking him to take on the roles of co-demon hunter and co-parent to Sammy. That was way too much for young Dean. Many folks IRL have experienced something similar.

Once you think of your own role in your family of origin, or first intimate social group, consider the roles of the other people in your family. Again, the intention is not to be judgmental or to blame anyone but simply to start to understand a bit more about yourself and how you came to be the superhero you are today. If you find that your core caregiver took on the role of "victim" in your family system, then it would make sense that one or more of the children would take on the role of caregiver.

Recall Storm's fanfic case study and her mention of her adoptive mother, Ainet. Part of Storm's struggle with her goddess role is linked to taking on the role of protector of both her adopted village and her adopted mother. They needed someone to cure the droughts that plagued their community, and, when Ororo (aka Storm) learned to control her mutant powers, she became a valued member of the community but with a price: treated as a teenage deity, Storm lost the chance to engage with her peers and progress through the developmental stages of adolescence. Another, albeit less charged, example of a parent as victim occurs in the beloved cartoon *Steven Universe*. Steven's hapless father is unable to care for his young son, Steven. Luckily, Steven has a triad of adopted mothers to intercede when Steven's father is unable to be the adult his son needs. Without the maternal power of the Crystal Gems, it is easy to imagine young Steven taking on the role of caregiver to his well-meaning but immature father. As you look at the different roles in your family of origin, you might notice such patterns.

Folks sometimes have a hard time wrapping their minds around the role of spousified child. People often ask us, "Are you talking about a literal child-bride type situation here?" And the answer is, no, though that would also apply. In its broadest definition, a spousified child refers to a child who has been given the role of co-parent or partner by one of the parents involved in the family system, usually following a crisis event that has changed the makeup of the family but not the needs of the system.[173] Some common crises are death, divorce, alcohol abuse, gambling, and affairs.

One of the best (or, worst) examples of spousification in fandom is that of Veronica and Keith Mars in the beloved cult classic television series *Veronica Mars*.[174] Veronica's mother walked out on the family, leaving an unfilled but needed role of partner. Veronica happily filled this role. While there are caregiving elements, Veronica is not a parentified child because she and her father relate as equals. The two work together, keep up their home, and share emotional burdens. This role can make it difficult for the spousefied child to eventually find a romantic partner, as time must be split between the romantic partner and the parent. The role can also inhibit parents from moving on emotionally, as they have a child to fill almost all needs in their life. Fans of the *Star Trek: Deep Space Nine* television series may find themselves considering whether Jake Sisko had a spousified relationship with his father.[175] After careful consideration, we'd argue that Commander Sisko does an excellent job of holding the line between supportive parent and thoughtful confidant. Great job, Sisko! Not only are you the Emissary to the Prophets and Commander of DS9, but you also kill it in the parenting department.

Closely related to the spousified child is the child-as-best-friend, which really is just what it sounds like. The *Gilmore Girls,* or a tale of two Lorelais, is arguably the most iconic example of parent and child as one another's best friend. In the WB television series, *Gilmore Girls*, Lorelai Gilmore gets pregnant as a teenager and gives birth to a daughter whom she names after herself: Lorelai Gilmore.[176] Fast forward fifteen years, and Lorelai and Lorelai, who now goes by Rory, are mother and daughter best friends living in the picturesque town of Stars Hollow. It all seems like fun and games (there's a lot of both), but Lorelai the elder's discomfort with the role of mother[lxiv] limits Rory's ability to differentiate herself from her mother and undermines Lorelai's ability to effectively teach and guide her daughter and seek out different kinds of fulfilling adult friendship.[lxv] The two reinforce the myth that single-parent homes are doomed to perpetuate unhealthy parent-child dynamics. Although the single-parent home often comes to mind, it is not the only system in which we find this dynamic. In fact, the child-as-best-friend dynamic runs rampant through the millennial child and boomer parent(s) family system.

Our final three roles take a look at the scapegoat, the golden child, and the problem child.[lxvi] This triad is linked to one of the great tenets of family therapy: nothing is personal; everything is systemic. In practice, this means that the roles assigned to family members may have little or nothing to do with the personality of the individual. But roles are always a result of the needs of the family system. The roles of scapegoat, golden child, and problem child can be (and often are) assigned to the children of the family, sometimes based entirely on the whims of birth order.

[lxiv] No doubt due to her tempestuous relationship with her own authoritarian mother, Emily Gilmore

[lxv] Hello, Luke Danes.

[lxvi] Woof.

Let's look at everyone's favorite cartoon family in *The Simpsons.*[177] Bart, the eldest, is most often the problem child and sometimes the scapegoat, a role he shares with his father, Homer. You might expect the eldest child to automatically take on the role of best and most-loved child, or golden child, but the Simpsons' system needs its first-born male child to attach to both parents without threatening them. Since neither Homer nor Marge are pillars of self-esteem and confidence, Bart is given the role of problem child, allowing both parents to dote on him without being at all threatened by him. Lisa, the second child, takes on the role of golden child in part because she is a girl and, thus, is far less threatening to her misogynistic father. For her mother, Lisa must hold all the deferred hopes and dreams Marge once had before she shackled herself to one Homer Simpson.[lxvii] Scapegoat is a role shared by Bart, Homer, and baby Maggie in large part because Bart and Homer are both prone to making messes, as is Maggie because she's, well, a baby and allowed to act her age because her elder siblings are doing so much emotional heavy lifting. Even in the most rigid families, the role of the scapegoat is often shared among the family members, though rarely at the same time. Anyone can be thrown under the family bus.

It might help to consider that roles arise out of necessity in the family system. The system becomes unbalanced in some way and the system wishes to rebalance.[178] Without insight, this balancing can look like the assigned roles of the Simpsons. These roles aren't assigned with mindful awareness, but they can be adjusted once they are acknowledged.

Reflecting on our past experiences in early social groups can stir up complicated feelings. Now might be a good time to pause and check in with your physical body. If you notice sweaty palms, elevated heart rate, shallow breathing, or fidgeting, this might indicate that it's time to take a break. Consider going for a walk, hydrating, or eating a nourishing meal or snack. Jefferson Starship will be here when you get back.

Are you feeling better? Wonderful, that's great to hear! You may ask yourself, *What was the point of all this anyway? Did we really need to psychoanalyze* The Simpsons*?* Well, here's the thing about our family of origin

---

[lxvii] RIP independent Marge.

roles: they have a *tremendous* impact on us when we become grown-up Yodas and head out into the world to form all manner of unique relationships: friendships, partnerships, companionships, etc. Or in the words of one of the founders of marriage and family therapy, Carl Whitaker, "Marriage is nothing but two scapegoats sent out into the forest to do battle over whose family system will be duplicated."[lxviii]

What Whitaker means is that the roles given to us in childhood inform how we show up in an adult relationship. Let's take a look at everyone's favorite *Star Trek: The Next Generation* couple,[lxix] Will Riker and Deanna Troi,[179] as an example. Deanna is the victim of spousification following the untimely death of her father. Her mother, Lwaxana Troi, is a charismatic and sexy figure who had a *lot* of romantic partners. Does this remind you of anyone? Yeah, exactly—Will Riker is also a charismatic and sexy figure who has a *lot* of romantic partners. Are we saying that Deanna married her mother? No, we're MFTs, not Freudians. We are saying that this early dynamic that Deanna has with a charismatic and sexually liberated person (i.e., her mother) teaches her how to be in a partnership with such a person. Will Riker has many attributes that Lwaxana does not have: he has a great beard, he's a loyal and caring friend, and, in general, he is respectful of boundaries.[lxx] For Deanna, Will Riker is the perfect combination of familiar and different.

Let's pause and reflect. Consider for a moment what roles you are drawn to in romantic relationships. Assess this versus the roles you held in your family of origin or first intimate social group. Remember to try to look at these without judgment; simply notice if you've brought some more old LEGO blocks into your grown-up life and whether you'd like to keep those classic toys or metaphorically donate some or all of them.

[lxviii] In our headcanon (and in the headcanon of our illustrious MFT professor Dr. Anne Ramage) this is how Carl said it. But you can find the actual quote in *The Family Crucible* (Napier and Whitaker, 1998/2017).

[lxix] No, not Wil Wheaton and Ashley Judd. Yes, Ashley Judd did star as a love interest for one, Wesley Crusher, and it was beautiful.

[lxx] A glaring exception is season 3, episode 14 of *The Next Generation*: "A Matter of Perspective."

Boundaries

At their simplest, boundaries are lines, sometimes visible and sometimes invisible, that separate us from other people or places. When we talk about boundaries within the context of systems, the term has a more nuanced meaning. Generally speaking, there are three types of boundaries: rigid, diffuse, and flexible.[180] Let's consider each type of boundary as if we were talking about a house. If you're a gamer, then you might think about the first house you own in *Stardew Valley*. Remember the two li'l windows, wooden door, and spacious grounds for gardening left to you by your uncle?[181] *Stardew Valley* is an excellent game for mindfulness, a topic we'll get into more in chapter 9 on screens, and it also serves as a helpful metaphor now as we talk about boundaries. In your mind's eye, picture your *Stardew Valley* house. If you aren't familiar with this house, then picture a compact brick house with two front-facing windows, a front door, a back door, and a garden surrounded by a waist-high fence. Roll with us; we promise it will make sense in a minute.

When you have rigid boundaries, both doors are locked, the blinds are drawn, and you've fortified your waist-high fence with concrete. Yeah, you're serious about the no-visitors sign affixed to your mailbox. The house is a closed system where nothing can get in and nothing can get out. It's a secure way to live, but it's also very lonely.

If you have diffuse boundaries, on the other hand, the windows and doors of your house are all open, as is the gate to even get into the yard. Nobody is vetting who or what is allowed in or out, so it's a free-for-all. The house is overrun with possums and raccoons, and nobody knows how they got in—they don't even realize they're allowed to shoo the wildlife back out. And when people and animals come and go, they bring and take emotions to the point that nobody really knows whose emotions belong to whom. It's chaotic and uncomfortable, but it has the illusion of openness and honesty.

Since this is a Goldilocks-type situation, you know that your goal is to have flexible boundaries: The doors and windows of your house are closed and locked, and the front gate is closed and latched. But the blinds are up, there's no fortified fence, and you've taken down that no-visitors sign because you are welcoming some visitors. With flexible boundaries, you get to decide who or what has access to the home that is you, and you have a choice of what visitors have to do to prove that they're safe to have on your property. By that we mean that you can choose to talk to your neighbors over the fence and never ask them to come into the yard. But maybe after you talk with your neighbor Pierre[lxxi] for a while and they show that they're trustworthy, you might invite them into the front yard. You do ask them to please not disturb the kale that you just planted. If they can respect that new boundary, then you might invite them onto the front porch. If they continue to prove themselves trustworthy, you might invite them into your foyer, as long as they are willing to remove their shoes. If, however, they are unwilling to remove their shoes and, additionally, they bring a raccoon with them, then you would direct them back out to the front stoop, the lawn, or maybe all the way onto the sidewalk.

Let's pause and take a breath. Now might be a good time to revisit your mind palace and take out your literal or metaphorical journal. We invite you to consider what type of boundaries your family of origin held. Did you feel like you had a choice in who came and went? Or did it feel like everybody was in each other's business? Or did it feel like nobody shared anything at all? Were there different rules based on the roles of the folks in the family? Remember to try to observe these memories without judgment, and perhaps jot this down so you don't forget. Now that you have an idea of what sorts of boundaries were in your family system, consider what types of boundaries you hold now in your romantic relationships. Are they similar or different? Neither answer is right or wrong. It's common to want to replay what you learned as a younger person, and it's also very common to leapfrog from diffuse to rigid or vice versa as you experiment doing things differently. As you reflect, tune in to your LEGO supply, and see if you'd like to set aside some boundary LEGOs for donation station.

After all three of these sections, you might find that you have a hefty pile of donation LEGOs; in fact, you might find that you have hardly any to keep at all. We invite you to pause and breathe. We challenge the idea that you have no LEGOs. Yes, you are deciding it's time to donate the old

---

[lxxi] We may never get over the fact that Pierre is not a marriageable character. It's almost as bad as Varric Tethras never being a romance option in the *Dragon Age* video game series.

LEGOs that no longer serve you, but if you turn to your metaphorical right, you might see a growing pile of shiny new LEGOS, ones you have chosen while reading this book and engaging in myriad positive IRL and fandom relationships throughout your journey. We invite you to reflect on some of these LEGOs and perhaps make a list of the positive rules, roles, and boundaries that you want to use as you build your LEGO bridge with your romantic partner(s).

The Trust Staircase

You may have noticed that the common thread that runs through the boundary section is about trust building. With flexible boundaries, we ensure that folks build trust before we allow them further access into our internal life. We tend to describe trust-building as a staircase: each time you set an expectation (don't touch my kale) and the other person respects that without you having to intervene, you move up a step on the trust staircase. If, however, the person does touch your kale or gets close to it and you say, "Hey, friend, remember the kale!" then you stay put on the staircase or move down a step. The goal in the trust staircase is to move up and down gradually and not wind up at the bottom of the staircase on your tuchus.

If you struggle with social anxiety like No-Face[182] from chapter 3, then you may feel pressure to rush up the trust staircase just to get the hard stuff out of the way. However, when you rush up the trust staircase, you don't pause to notice how your potential romantic partner treated your kale patch or whether or not they took off their shoes like you asked in the foyer. Also, remember that you are not the only person on the trust staircase. It isn't just about them building trust with you, but also you are building trust with them. It's important to be mindful of the other stair-climber's wants and needs.

Communication

In our work with clients around rules, roles, and boundaries, we often hear the following questions: "How do I actually have tough conversations about boundaries with other people?" "How do I know whether another human is really trustworthy and won't hurt me like other people in my life have?" The short answer is that we can never truly know what another person is going to do. However, when we engage with other humans in a way that helps us to build trust over time, we are giving the other person the opportunity to show us who they are. Sometimes we just don't like what we see.

For example, imagine that you're meeting a new potential friend for the first time. Did that spark anxiety? That's fair. Take a breath. Let's start again. Imagine that you are meeting a potential friend for the first time and you want to begin to move up the trust staircase with them. If you currently hold diffuse boundaries, you might think, *I'm going to tell them every single thing that I've been through in life and everything that I'm going through now so that they know what they're getting into. If they hear all that and run, then I'll know what kind of person they really are.* Whoa, friend. We get the inclination. But diffuse boundaries really aren't fair to you or your potential new friend because you're asking them to hold top-of-the-staircase information before you've even gone up one step. This type of boundarylessness is another form of pushing people away so that you can walk away from the situation feeling like you tried. Conversely, if you hold rigid boundaries, you might be resistant to tell your new potential friend anything at all about yourself. Unfortunately, it's nearly impossible to form a relationship that way.

As mimicking creatures, we want to experience a similar amount of disclosure back and forth. So how about we start this possible new friendship with a mild disclosure, like a fandom that you're into?

For example, you say you're into *Doctor Who*, and, hey, so are they! How great! Then you might take your disclosure a bit further and say that your favorite doctor is Nine. If they make a face and say, "Um, actually, Ten is far superior," then you might not want to make any more disclosures right now. But if they say "yeah, Nine's cool. Ten is definitely *my* doctor, though," then maybe you take a step up the staircase. Did you pick up on the subtle distinction between those two answers? In the first one, your potential new friend is making a judgment about something that you like. If they can't handle your doctor preference, how are they going to handle your trauma history? But in the second one, the new friend shows that they can accept a difference of opinion without it being a personal attack. Lots of folks in the world of fandom could learn the importance of this distinction.

OK, you say to yourself, *that's fine for a new friendship, but what about a potential romantic relationship? Surely that's a different story, right?* Nope! You go through the same process whether you're making platonic or romantic partnerships. The bottom line is that you need to trust the other human in the relationship, and the way that you do that is through mild disclosures followed by slightly larger disclosures that are accepted and are then reciprocated by the other party, slowly taking step after step up the staircase.

Once you've built trust and find yourself in a relationship, the communication doesn't stop there. Once trust is established, it can be helpful to assume neutral-to-positive intent in most interactions. This doesn't mean that you just let it go when your partner says or does something that feels hurtful. Rather, reminding yourself of neutral-to-positive intent can help you shift to a place of internal curiosity from which to initiate a discussion. For example, when Eliot offers Margo a drink from his never-ending flask, Margo could assume negative intent, such as *Eliot thinks I need a drink to calm down*, or she could assume neutral-to-positive intent, such as *Maybe Eliot wants to comfort me over drinks.* Margo can then pause and check in with herself to notice how she's feeling. Then, she can decide to verbally initiate a clarifying conversation or continue on with their hike in the Fillorian wilds.

Hogwarts Personality Types

Relationships are all about communication. Yet even when we understand our partner's perspective, it can be difficult when it feels like our romantic partner or partners don't see things the way that we do. The great news is that the concept of perfect compatibility is a myth! Similar to the concept of posttraumatic growth, discussed in chapter 4, we can grow and develop our compatibility with another person provided that they and we are willing to do the work. Lots of successful pairings occur between quite different humans who learn how to live together. Think of Sherlock and John,[183] Dean and Castiel, or *Star Trek: Discovery*'s Michael and Ash the transmogrified human formerly known as the Klingon Voq.[184] The same is true out in the real world.

A great way to think about personality differences is in terms of Hogwarts Houses.[lxxii] Each Hogwarts House has a certain personality trait that they prize above all others. Gryffindor house prizes bravery, Slytherin prizes cunning, Hufflepuff prizes loyalty, and Ravenclaw prizes wisdom. Knowing that you are a Ravenclaw and your partner is a Hufflepuff gives you valuable information about what they prize and how they see the world. If you're having an argument, as a Ravenclaw, it might be most important to you to have the right answer, and you might want to do research to back up your point of view, whereas your partner might be most focused on preserving your relationship, regardless of the facts of the argument. You can see how this could keep a fight going. The Ravenclaw would be frustrated that their research isn't being respected, and the Hufflepuff would be frustrated that the Ravenclaw keeps throwing out facts instead of meeting them on an emotional level to make things better. Neither perspective is right or wrong; they just highlight the different ways people can approach problems. As you and your partner become aware of these differences, your compatibility grows.

Initially, couples notice how differently they react and might interpret this as negative. The Hufflepuff sees themselves as trying to build the relationship and sees their partner Ravenclaw as trying to keep fighting. But once partners begin to understand the other's point of view, they can start to see the world through the other's eyes and thus more correctly interpret the other's actions. So the Hufflepuff can begin to see that the Ravenclaw isn't trying to fight; the Ravenclaw is trying to show their Hufflepuff partner that the relationship is very important. It's worth their time and effort to engage wisdom, their most important aspect.

Hogwarts Houses can also help you to understand your own and your partner's preferred forms of attachment communication. What we're referring to here are all the ways that an individual verbally and nonverbally seeks care and expresses care to their romantic partner. For those of you

---

[lxxii] Finding out what Hogwarts House your partner belongs to is another possible early disclosure to share.

acquainted with the five love languages, this might all sound a bit familiar.[185] As with so many psychological concepts, we have taken what works for us and fanficced the rest. But if you're a Ravenclaw who wants to know about the original five love languages, they are Words of Affirmation, Acts of Service, Receiving/Giving Gifts, Quality Time, and Physical Touch.[186]

Slytherins are known for their cunning, ambition, shrewdness, and independence. They tend to seek out situations in which they can be publicly recognized for achievement and tend to prefer working alone rather than in groups. Slytherins have a strong sense of self-preservation, which means that if they feel like their self or their livelihood is being threatened, they are prone to going full dracarys.[lxxiii] In a partnership, Slytherins tend to appreciate lots of verbal affirmation. This isn't to say that they don't appreciate loving acts, but they need their partners to explain and verbally name these loving acts if said partner wants to get laid.

Hufflepuffs are often associated with plants, snacks, and creatures of all kinds. They also tend to value hard work, dedication, patience, loyalty, and fairness. Hufflepuffs tend to sit in the middle on the introvert-extrovert spectrum, which helps to explain why they tend to feel nearly equal appreciation for loving, loyal, or caring actions shown toward themselves as toward their friends. Hufflepuffs tend to have very tender hearts that are easily bruised. If you are partnered with a Hufflepuff, care needs to be taken in how you express your words. A Hufflepuff may react negatively to loud expressions of anger even if that anger is not directed at them but, say, at a particular external event.

Ravenclaws are the cleverest, wittiest, and smartest of witches. We aren't saying that this is our house. But clearly it is. Ravenclaws appreciate kind, smart, and funny words, particularly when written with grammatical and spelling accuracy. They are also pleased when acts of service are done for them, such as bringing them tea or returning their overdue book to the library. They tend to prefer expressing affection with words and shared enjoyment of quality time reading together. Sherlock is a classic Ravenclaw who has to negotiate relationship rules with his Gryffinpuff[lxxiv] partner John.

[lxxiii] *Dracarys* is the *Game of Thrones* term for burning it all down.

[lxxiv] Hybrids of houses definitely exist!

Gryffindors are kind of the worst. Just kidding! We love you, Gryffindors. If you are a Gryffindor, you may feel a bit upset right now, even though we very quickly explained that we were joking. While Gryffindors are often courageous, daring, and chivalrous, they also tend to struggle with being both reckless and short-tempered. The good news here is that they tend to cool off pretty quickly. So by the time they've made it to this sentence, they might even have forgiven us for our bad joke! One of our favorite fandom examples of a Gryffindor (besides Harry, Ron, and Hermione) is Han Solo. Han loved to show off in front of Leia almost as much as he loved flirtatious banter.

What do you do when your partner is a hybrid? Well, the best thing is to be curious, using verbal communication to explore what parts of them resonate with Gryffindor and what parts resonate with Hufflepuff, for example. There are no right or wrong answers, just new information that you both can use to grow compatibility, such as understanding how to make up after arguments, show and express affection, and negotiate chores (ugh, like vacuuming). No matter how much you love your partner, you probably don't love cleaning up your shared space—unless you're a Ravenpuff, in which case then you might just love it! You might notice that this chapter was clearly written by two Ravenclaws (so many different definitions).

You might feel a little overwhelmed by how much early familial experiences impact your romantic relationship dynamics as an adult (more on this in the next chapter). Wherever you're at, we invite you to take a moment to consider the following: Romance[lxxv] isn't easy. But with some introspection, active reflection, and study, you can learn the spells and skills to keep yourself safe and playful on the broom ride of romance.

[lxxv] Romeo and Juliet? Edward and Bella? Heathcliff and Cathy? Storm and Black Panther? Scott, Jean, and Wolverine?

FANFIC CASE STUDY:
The Magicians, Family and Further

Though we certainly enjoyed our sojourn in Lawrence, Kansas—Dean's apple pie never disappoints—we knew it was time to depart. Having received an invitation from our dear friend Dean Fogg, we decamp for Brakebills University, where we plan to teach for two semesters as visiting professors. Happy to put our therapizing aside for a time and take up the gauntlet of teaching, we ought to have known better than to think our reputations would do anything but precede us. It isn't but a fortnight until a new client—or more precisely a new couple—grace our doorstep asking for help.

The storm howls outside as we doze in our offices upon twin plush settees next to a roaring fire in the fireplace. Suddenly, we hear the sounds of voices and an abrupt banging at our door.

"Jesus fucking Christ, Eliot!" booms a voice.

"Bambi!" responds another.

Before we can get to the door, a burst of air, a clash of lightning, and the stench of burning rubber all happen simultaneously as the door to our offices crashes down to reveal the two human magicians in question: Margo Hanson and Eliot Waugh.

Eliot, impeccably attired and with curls only slightly damp, steps over the door and into our offices. Turning to his equally well-dressed companion he asks, "Was that really necessary?"

"Yeah, it *was*. We've been together for at least the human equivalent of over a dozen lifetimes, and I'm not letting your depression destroy us. We survived the Beast remember? We brought you back from that depraved dimension house in the ancient god's house-of-horrors head." With a toss of her head and flick of her wrist, Margo dispatches her velvet-trimmed riding cloak—a deep navy with emerald trim—and sets the door back on its hinges.

"Bambi!" exclaims the objectively handsome magician.

"What?" retorts his equally majestic companion.

"Your powers of alliteration really have improved!"

Margo's red lips part into a smile. "I know." She takes the hand that Eliot offers her and leads him into our offices. Standing before the fire, the two survey the room, and Eliot makes a noise between a cough and a sigh.

"How *sad*. You don't seem to have enough chairs."

"Well, we didn't plan to see clients at Brakebills," we answer.

"Clients? Please. We'll only need one session. If you're as good as Link says, you'll have us fixed up in no time."

We glance at each other in surprise: "You know the hero of Hyrule?"

Eliot shakes out his chestnut locks and slowly cracks the knuckle of his left thumb. Barely glancing at us, he replies, "Honestly, Jefferson Starship. We know everyone."

We chuckle to ourselves and mutter under our breaths, "That nickname really has some staying power."

"Stand back, please," Eliot advises, and we only have time to look up before Eliot's long pale fingers contort and twist themselves in positions that can only be described as hand yoga. He mutters something in Turkish, or possibly Sanskrit.

"Weren't you *listening*?" Margo cries as she grabs both our arms and jerks us back just in time for a large golden plush sofa to crash down to the carpet where moments before we had been standing. Margo rolls her eyes at us and dusts off her hands. "Beautiful job, E." She leans over and kisses him fondly. "But red instead of yellow, I think?"

"Your wish is my command," and with one final wrist flick, the upholstery is changed to a tone befitting two former high kings of Fillory.

"Your majesties," we curtly bow before taking our own seats—one in either armchair—and face the couple before us. "How can we be of help?"

Margo smiles satisfactorily. "See? I told you they'd see us."

"Apologies," begins Eliot, as he accepts the tea we offer him, "it's my understanding that you were on something of a therapeutic sabbatical."

We shrug. "Those don't seem to last long for us."

"Well, a gift's a gift" Margo breezes, "Now, let's get down to business, shall we? Eliot here is depressed, and you need to fix him."

"Bambi, you know feelings don't work that way."

"No, I certainly don't. That's why I'm here, consulting with the experts." She gestures to us as she pulls out a crystal dropper.

"May we ask what that is?"

She furrows her brow. "Fairy dust."

"As a general rule, we ask that you not imbibe mind-altering substances during session."

Margo guffaws loudly.

"As you say, we are the experts in emotions. And for us to be helpful to you, you need to be fully capable of connecting with your feelings, as it feels safe to do so."

"As a general rule, I like to keep myself to two emotions at once. One I'm feeling and one I'm hiding," Margo replies.

"That's very honest of you."

Margo puts the crystal dropper away, storing it within the recesses of her raven-colored tunic. "Not going to do much good here if I'm lying."

We shift our gaze to Eliot. His eyes have become wet.

"You really are worried about me."

"Of course I'm worried!" Margo snaps. "You barely talk to me. When I send rabbits from Fillory, you don't respond—not to jokes, not to gossip, not even to the verbal sex picture I sent."

Eliot's mouth turns upward in the slightest hint of a smile. "That was very inventive."

"You see what I'm dealing with here?" Margo gestures, sparks flying from her bejeweled fingertips.

"What is your relationship to one another exactly?" we ask, looking from one to the other then back again.

"We're lovers," intones Eliot.

"He's my best friend," says Margo.

"We met at Brakebills," Margo begins, leaning into the arm that Eliot puts behind her head.

"We weren't exactly fast friends."

"More like low-key adversaries."

"Frenemies?"

"Honey, I didn't even know your name."

"Ouch," Eliot laughs, his first real smile of the session. "Yes, well, we got teamed up together for trials."

"We fuckin' wasted the rest of those nerds."

"And then we fucked like rabbits."

"Our first orgy," Margo smiles, lacing her right hand through Eliot's left. Eliot closes his eyes, tips back his head, and smiles. In a matter of seconds, it shifts to a grimace.

"Those were the days," he finishes sadly.

"See, this is the problem right here, Docs."

"We aren't—"

"I know, I know, but who cares? A title only gets power if you give it. I was High King of Fillory. Was that grammatically correct? Who gives a fuck? So, Docs, here's my problem. Just now we were about to have a nice reverie that usually leads to at least hand stuff—"

Eliot smiles again: "Please, Bambi, at least a threesome."

"Exactly. But instead he cuts it off with his doom-and-gloom shit and ends up moaning about Quentin."

At this, Eliot disentangles himself from Margo, the leader formerly known as High King Margo, and retreats to the opposite end of the couch. "It hasn't even been a year."

"In Fillory time it's been five," Margo retorts, folding her arms across her chest.

"Well, I don't live in Fillory."

"Only because you've chosen not to. I've invited you—"

"And what would I do there? Watch as you and Josh gallivant around like husband and wife while I sit in the corner and fondle the fawns? Consensually, of course," Eliot adds when he looks up and sees the concern on our faces.

Margo lays her hands facing up in her lap. "Eliot, I'm sorry. I miss him too. You know I do."

"It's not the same for you," Eliot replies, staring into the fire.

Margo looks away to the shadows playing darts in the corner. "No, it's not."

"What happened to Quentin?" We ask.

"He died," they both intone together.

"He was my husband."

"He was his husband." They each say, almost simultaneously.

"Or he was at least in another life." Eliot grips a pillow, a sound catching in his throat.

"And he probably would have been again if he'd lived," Margo finishes, lifting a hand and letting it hover above Eliot's back.

"Have you let yourself cry?" we inquire.

"Oh, my gods, are you serious? All he does is cry."

"No, not Eliot, Margo. You. Have you let yourself cry?"

Margo turns to face us fully, her left hand shaking slightly. "What do you mean?"

"Have you cried for the loss you have suffered?"

"I didn't love Quentin like that. He was my friend, but..." Margo looks down at her hands. "He wasn't my partner. Not even Josh is my partner. Eliot is my partner. And I'm losing him."

"Does part of you fear that you already have?" We ask.

Margo's face crumples. "Fuck you."

Eliot drops the pillow. He turns toward Margo. "Bambi?"

She begins to cry, mascara bleeding down her face in two black rivulets.

"Is that true?"

Between sobs, Margo says, "Eliot, you're not the same since Quentin died. I know how important he was to you—more important than Josh is to me. And you know how much I love banging Josh."

Eliot nods. "If the rumors are to be believed, it's a whole fucking lot."

Through her tears, Margo smiles. "And it never bothered me. No, honestly, it didn't. You and Q. I never felt threatened by him and you. I knew what you meant to each other. I wasn't surprised when you came back after you lived that whole lifetime to solve that puzzle spell and said you felt married to him. Honestly, I was more surprised that you two didn't make it official."

"It's my greatest regret," Eliot answers, reaching out for Margo's hand. Margo closes her fingers around Eliot's right hand while she lifts her right to wipe the mascara away.

"Figures I'd choose the unenchanted kind today," she laughs.

"You do look a complete mess," Eliot affirms.

"I love you, Eliot."

"I love you too, Bambi. I don't want this to change."

"But how could it not change?" We ask the couple as they turn to look at us. "From the sounds of it, you and your friends have lived multiple lifetimes on various different worlds. You've changed as individuals, so of course your relationship to one another is going to change."

Margo begins to cry again, this time softly. "But I don't want us to change. We've always been each other's constant."

Eliot turns fully toward Margo and takes both her hands in his. "Maybe it doesn't have to be a bad change. Maybe it's just an acknowledgment of what has happened to us. It can deepen what we have."

"You do know I like it deep."

"I know," Eliot smiles, lifting a hand to shift a tendril of hair from Margo's eyelashes.

"We're not gonna be done in one session, are we?"

"No," we answer the couple, "we don't think that was ever an option. But with several months of work, we can help the two of you process your individual grieving and learn different ways to support each other. And continue to grow and change in a way that leads you back together rather than far apart."

"I'd like that," Margo says, tightening her grip around Eliot's hands. "What do you think, E?"

"Oh, I called ahead—last week. And booked us for weekly sessions for the next three months."

"You motherfucker," Margo laughs, gently pulling her hands away. "I've gotta do something with this face. We can't be seen out in Brakebills looking like Brangelina circa 2016."

"Oh, Bambi, on our worst day we're better than those two muggles at their *Mr. & Mrs. Smith* hottest."

Margo smiles.

FANFIC CASE STUDY QUESTIONS:
We Invite You to Answer Some Fucking Magical Questions

- Describe some of the relational groups in which Margo and Eliot are involved. How do they use verbal communication to help navigate these different systems while remaining close to one another?
- In what ways could Margo and Eliot benefit from more clearly defined boundaries in their current relational dynamic?
- Who in your life has been challenging to set boundaries with? How might you engage them in a dialogue around this struggle?

YOGA:
Hand Magic

If you are in *The Magician*'s fandom, you're no stranger to the yogic hand magic that they use. This practice can be done anywhere and anytime and is for conjuring energy, introspection, and collaboration. Feel free to practice poses one at a time slowly, or speed up and do your best magician impression.

Begin seated or standing, whichever feels better to you. This spell isn't reliant on your foot position. Pause here and take a couple breaths to get centered before practicing your magic.

1. Heart Pose: Bring your hands together, palms touching, with your thumbs touching the center of your sternum. This position will be where the spells begin and end, and you will return to it between each of the other poses.

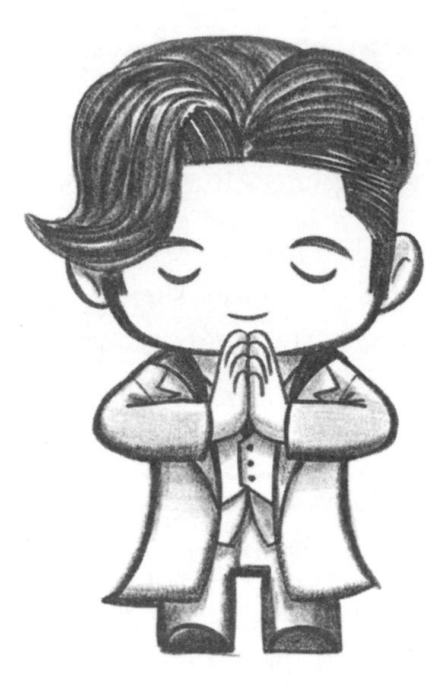

2. Removing Wards Pose: Starting from Heart Pose, twist your hands so that your fingers face your opposite wrists. Slide your fingers so that you can clasp them together with your opposite hand. Clasp them tightly.

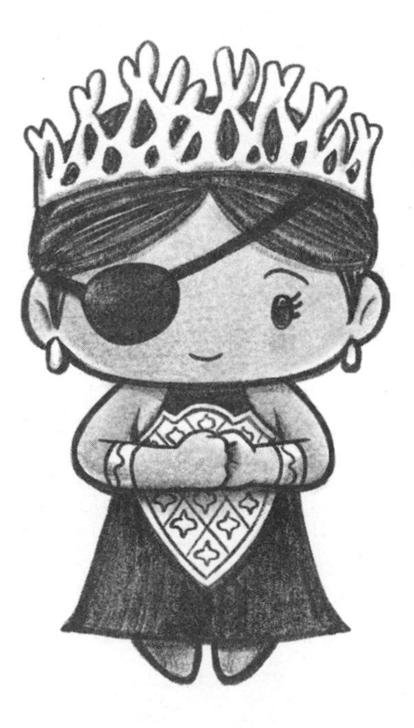

3. Return to your Heart Pose.
4. High King Margo Pose: From Heart Pose, interlace all ten fingers, and then release your index finger creating a steeple grip. Point your steeple forward with conviction.

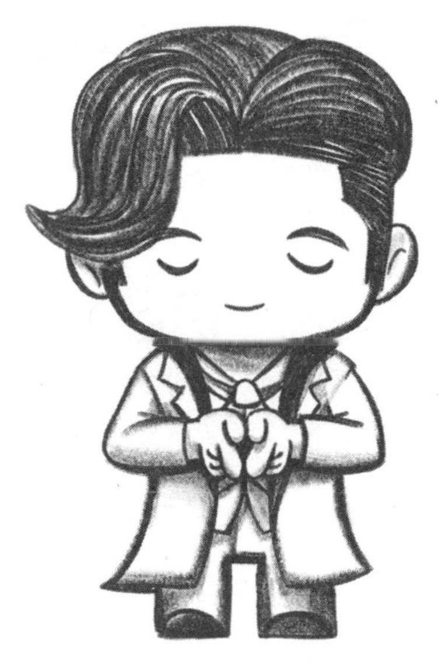

5. Return to your Heart Pose.
6. Fillorian Sage Pose: Place the back of your right hand on top of your left palm so that palms face upward, and touch your thumbs together. Pause here, and allow the Fillorian sages to calm you.

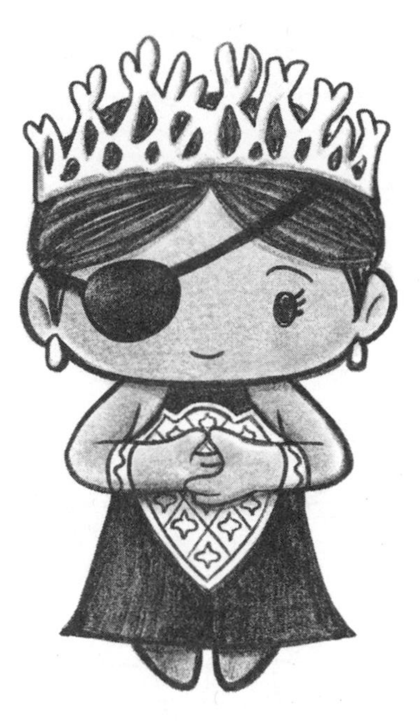

7. Return to your Heart Pose.
8. High King Eliot Pose: With the elegance of Eliot, bring your hands in front of you at about shoulder height, palms facing forward. Bring your index and ring finger to touch your thumb on each hand.

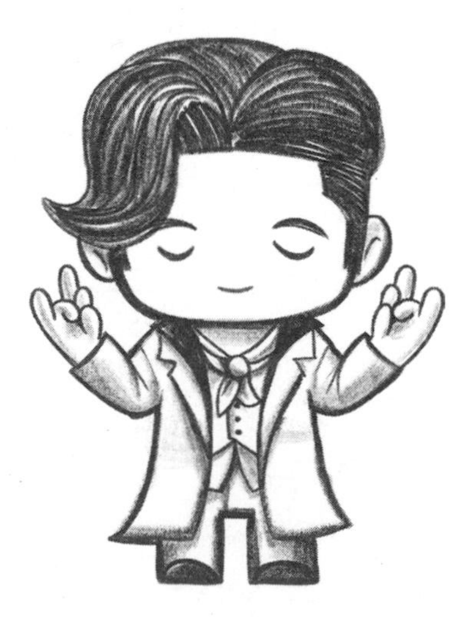

9. Return to your Heart Pose.
10. Unshakable Trust Pose: From your Heart Pose, interlace your fingers and release your thumbs. With the ferocity that only Margo can bring, forcefully press the backs of your hands forward.

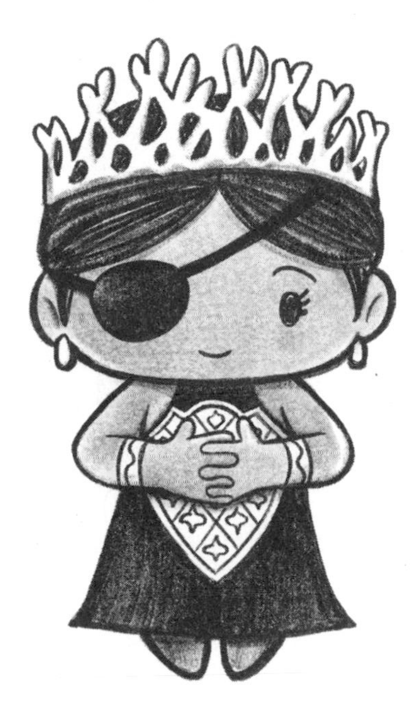

11. Return to your Heart Pose.

The Trouble with Family

Family don't end with blood.

—BOBBY, ***SUPERNATURAL***, "NO REST FOR THE WICKED"[187]

Families, our first social groups or systems, play a huge role in how we show up in our lives. Human beings are social creatures, which means we learn how to be a human being by watching and then imitating the humans around us.[188] We inherit some of our first stories from our first intimate social group or family of origin. Knowing a little bit more about families is helpful not just in romantic relationships but also on our journey to identify and then change the stories that no longer serve us. With this knowledge we can really level up those Therapeutic Fanfiction skills.

Transgenerational Wiccans, Wakandans, and Mice

The Wicked + The Divine comic series charts the rebirth of a group of gods in the twenty-first century. They have been reincarnated numerous times, and most of them don't have chronological memory of their past selves or incarnations.[189] Rather, they have emotion-based memory that pops up at generally inopportune moments during times of crisis. If this sounds a lot like trauma memory, that's because it is. Or, to be most precise, this is transgenerational trauma in action.

Transgenerational trauma is both encoded in our genetics and modeled by our family of origin, and it impacts us on emotional and physical[190] levels, even though we, just like *The Wicked + The Divine* gods, don't have a fact-based memory to which this emotion-based memory is attached.[191] This explains the confusion folks may have felt as children when they knew something wasn't quite right in their family of origin but couldn't put their finger on what that something was.[192]

Maybe you remember feeling like your core caregiver just wasn't able to attach to you the way that you saw other parents connecting with their kids. One of the reasons could be transgenerational trauma. When parents have experienced a trauma, they can give that shittily wrapped epigenetic gift to their kids. But beyond genetics, when folks have experienced trauma, it also impacts their affect, or the way that they interact and show up with others.[193] Sometimes you receive these gifts from long ago. These traumas can be personal tragedies experienced by the family[194] as well as cultural traumas experienced by a group of people. Those of African descent who experienced the horrors of slavery, colonization, and systemic oppression pass this trauma on to their children and future generations.[195] Evidence suggests that people with relatives who were in the Holocaust "remember" that experience.[196]

Now let's explore two examples of transgenerational trauma through fandom in the *Black Panther* film and comic series and the graphic novel *Maus*. We invite you to please take care of your self: mind, body, and fandom. If you need to take breaks or skip this section entirely, please know that you can definitely do so.

Both T'Challa and N'Jadaka (aka Erik Stevens, aka Killmonger), the hero and antihero of the *Black Panther* franchise, struggle with transgenerational trauma.[197] T'Challa grapples with the transgenerational trauma of the African continent's colonization. T'Challa's father directly communicates to his son the horrors of colonialism witnessed by previous Wakandan kings. T'Challa himself is often depicted as having a visceral reaction or trauma response when the idea of opening Wakanda's borders is first broached in both the comic and cinematic iterations.[198] N'Jadaka has a different experience of transgenerational trauma because his mother is African American.[lxxvi] In addition to his father's (N'Jobu's) genetic trauma and the written journal of memories he leaves for his son, N'Jadaka's mother passes on to him the traumas of slavery and the marginalization and systemic oppression that African American folks experienced in the new world. As we discussed in chapter 4, N'Jadaka's and T'Challa's legacy of trauma informs their relationship with one another and the world. Perhaps because T'Challa has words for the transgenerational trauma he inherits, he is able to engage in posttraumatic growth. Orphaned and abandoned by his Wakandan family,[199] N'Jadaka is denied the connection and language that might have helped him process his personal and transgenerational trauma.[200]

A great and also terrible (meaning difficult) example of this is in the graphic novel *Maus,* which depicts the author, Art Spiegelman, interviewing his father, Vladek, about World War II.[201] The author portrays the events in the camps and his family's journey through them before he was born. The reader gets the benefit of experiencing both Art and Vladek's experiences. In *Maus*, Vladek never really returns from the war. There were too many losses, too much trauma, too much change. Perhaps most impactful, Vladek's son, Art's would-be older brother, Richieu, doesn't survive the war. Similar to Sethe's decision in Toni Morrison's literary classic *Beloved* to kill her children to prevent them from growing up in slavery,[202] Art's elder brother is the victim of a mercy killing by his caretakers to prevent him from going to the camps. (We recognize this is a lot of trauma. Again, please take your time with it.) Through the interview process, Art comes to see how his father became a man who refuses to throw away one slip of paper, seemingly more attached to a broken plate than to his own son. Like T'Challa, Art gets the language that he needs to reframe, label, and finally understand both his own trauma and the trauma of his forebears.

[lxxvi] In the *Black Panther* film.

Though you might have experienced transgenerational trauma in your family, it doesn't mean that you're doomed. Although your genes will continue to express this experience, nurture is a powerful ally of nature and can foster healing change no matter how old or young you are.[203] If you choose to do things differently and heal from the trauma, you can have a different experience, as can all of those with whom you are or wish to be attached.[204] Now might be a good time to recall, if not straight-up revisit, chapter 4 on posttraumatic growth and its tips and tricks for such a healing journey. First and foremost, identifying the pain you have inherited transgenerationally and via parental modeling can move you forth on this path. In our work as therapists, this is the point in our journey with folks that we often introduce the genogram, or therapy family tree, to help. A genogram is a pictorial representation of a person and the family groups that raised and/or influenced them.[205] Although the genogram is based on the concepts and theories of Murray Bowen,[lxxvii] it was fully developed and made popular by Bowenian theorists Monica McGoldrick and Randy Gerson. Behold the Spiegelman family tree, complete with trauma both in the present and inherited past:

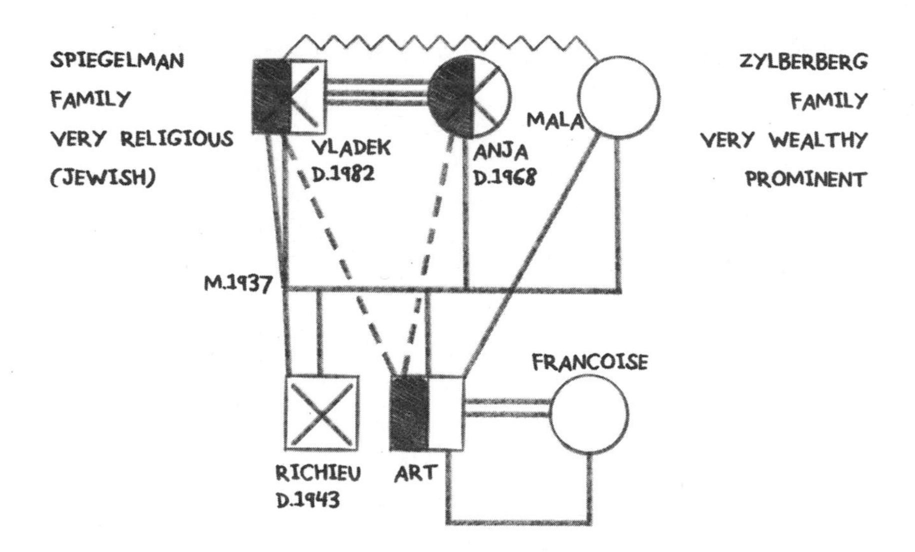

[lxxvii] Murray is basically the grandfather of marriage and family therapy, or the paterfamilias, if you will. More on him later.

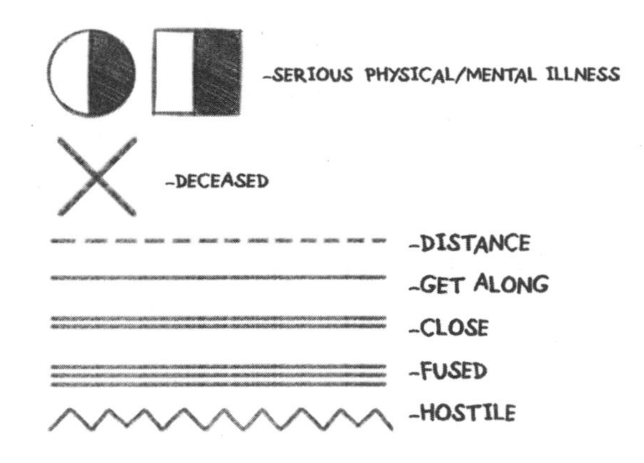

As you can see, genograms allow us to understand a bit about how we came to be who we are and how our parents became who they are or were, and on and on. Learning about the pain of past generations does not excuse anyone's behavior but simply helps us to understand and hopefully come to a sense of peace about the past.[206] In this genogram you find the Spiegelman and Zylberberg families. The Spiegelmans are very religious and find comfort in their Judaism. Vladek's faith would become a protective factor for him in the camps. The Zylberbergs were very wealthy; Vladek describes them as millionaires. His joining with his wife Anja changed his life circumstances considerably, as he was given a high-status job from his high-status father-in-law. Vladek's life might've looked very different had he not married Anja. The Zylberbergs go on to lose everything in the war. Even before the war, Anja experiences serious and persistent mental illness and spends time in a facility, where Vladek lives with her—something that would be impossible for someone of less means. Vladek and Anja's child, Richieu, was doted upon by the entire family. Richieu's loss was excruciating. Long after the end of WWII, when Art is an adult, his mother ends her own life without leaving a note. Her mental illness was exacerbated by all that she experienced. Art also deals with mental illness, for which he is briefly institutionalized. Vladek could not move past the loss of Anja because of how fused (or enmeshed) their relationship was (more on enmeshment in a bit). Vladek does remarry a woman named Mala, whom he does not like. They fight incessantly, and he's convinced that she's going to steal all his money.

Vladek deals with a great deal of physical illness and eventually starts to lose grasp of reality due to dementia.

This is a difficult story and also an important one. We walk through the genogram a bit so that you can see, particularly for Vladek, how his experiences shape the ways he interacts with his loved ones. He worked tirelessly to build relationships with his "first family": Anja, Richieu, and his extended in-laws. The war destroys all those connections. With his "second family" composed of Art and Mala, Vladek builds weak connections, easily broken and easily mourned.

Knives Out Grandpa Bowen: My House, My Rules, My Coffee

We promised you more on Murray Bowen, and here it is. Bowen introduced one of our favorite concepts in the field of marriage and family therapy: differentiation.[207] Remember back in the last chapter when we talked about rules, roles, and boundaries? These principles will serve you well in understanding this concept. The goal of differentiation is finding the boundary "sweet spot" with your family of origin so that you are both separate and connected with them. That is, you are neither cut off with no contact nor so enmeshed that you can't tell where your stuff ends and your family's stuff begins.[208] No doubt, Grandpa Murray would have had a lot to say about the Thrombey clan, an eccentric WASPy family depicted in the film *Knives Out* that lives off the fame and fortune of the titular patriarch.[209] Perhaps most glaringly, this family is in desperate need of some differentiation. They're so enmeshed and dependent upon their aging paterfamilias that they can't imagine a life without him. Although we take issue with some of Harlan Thrombey's methods, we tend to agree with his assessment that his children and grandchildren each needed to set out on their own respective hero's journeys.[lxxviii]

[lxxviii] And we also tend to agree that Harlan had his own unquestioned reasons for keeping his family so dependent on him. There's nothing like being needed to help you feel like a hero.

Let's pause for a moment and review your journaling. What did you discover about your boundaries with your family of origin? If you found that you're on one of the extremes, consider what it would be like to be both separate and connected to your family. Sometimes it isn't safe to have an in-person connection at all, and we get that. But consider, even if you don't engage with your family, whether they take up emotional space in your mind. If they do, then you might not be quite as cut off as you think you are.

What about family roles?[210] Did you discover that your early family of origin role was similar to Lorelai Gilmore in relationship to Emily, or are you more of a Rory?[lxxix] Or perhaps you identified with the spousified Veronica Mars. Relatedly, there's the experience of Steven, Storm, and Dean, who were all parentified by at least one of their original family systems. And perhaps some of you journaled about experiences with your own personal Mando. Whatever roles you realized in your journaling related to chapter 7, now is a great time to reflect on it in the context of this idea of differentiation. Which, if any, of the roles you were given as a child still resonate for you? You may find that some of the roles still work or that you've found ways to repurpose them so that they feel more resonant to your adult self. Storm finds ways to repurpose some of the skills learned during her childhood experiences of parentification for her chosen role as co-leader of the X-Men. Or perhaps a past traumatic experience can be used to help you better understand a present moment and to make meaning. Mando of the *The Mandalorian* is an excellent example of a person who suffers an incredible trauma: watching the Empire annihilate his parents and home planet. He uses this event to empathize and then connect with Baby Yoda, eventually making new meaning from his trauma when he fully commits to his new role as guardian and parent to the Child, Grogu.

Finally, review your journaling and/or reflect on your musings related to rules during chapter 7. We invite you to reflect now on the rules that you identified in your family of origin and the ways those rules inform your life today. Recall the time we spent in session with Dean Winchester. If you apply what you learned in chapter 7, it's easy to see that he grew up with

---

[lxxix] And for the record, we just are not even touching season 8 of *Gilmore Girls*. No hate to those of you who loved it; we just didn't.

the following rules: Don't ask for help. Don't show weakness. Take care of Sammy. Don't complain. Always have rock salt on hand. Use classic rock to scream out any of the feelings you aren't able to repress. Dean carries these rules with him into adulthood and, thus, regularly struggles to ask for help and to let that one man-tear fall. But just because you were given a rule, or a role, or a certain type of boundary when you were young does not mean you have to carry it forth into your adult life. No, friends. Just like Dean and Storm, you can rewrite your internal script. You can use the tools of Therapeutic Fanfiction to change your life. Or in the spirit of Carl Whitaker, what you don't pass back you pass forward. What Whitaker means here is that you do not have to keep every rule, role, boundary, and tool given to you by the previous generation. Instead, you can decide what still resonates with you and what doesn't. All that stuff in the "no longer applicable LEGO pile" can be passed back to gramps and gran.

This brings us all the way back around to differentiation. In order to differentiate, we must reflect, review, and then revise some or all of the rules, roles, and boundaries that connect us to our families of origin. For the Jungians out there, differentiation can be confused with individuation or the process by which parts of the unconscious become conscious via a long series of therapeutic confrontations between an individual's unconscious and conscious minds.[211]

If you are a Jungian or just a fan of the Jung-infused *Control* video game, it might be helpful to think of differentiation as the systemic version of individuation. Through a series of renegotiations with the individual and their family of origin over time, the individual learns new ways to actualize while renegotiating and creating new attachment dynamics with their family of origin. And who exemplifies this better than the crew of *The Expanse*?[212]

Whether you are a fan of the television show or of the book series, or you simply tolerate your best friend's undying love for both, you can probably already start to see the interpersonal dynamics we've discussed playing out in the chosen family of the *Rocinante* starship: Amos, an Earther mechanic with a traumatic past,[213] learns how to connect with and trust his *Roci* shipmates by using the tools of posttraumatic growth. Alex, a Martian deadbeat dad, learns how to accept himself and take responsibility for his past transgression through the support of his shipmates and his successful role as the pilot of the *Roci.*[214] Though she presents as the most "together" of the crew, Naomi, a Belter engineer, has struggles of her own that lead to secret keeping,[215] thereby limiting her shipmates' ability to show up for her. Holden, captain of the *Roci,* renegotiates his boundaries and role within his polyamorous family of origin—he's got three mothers and five fathers in what is known in *The Expanse* universe as a marriage co-op—thanks to the support of his romantic life partner, Naomi.[216] When we first meet Holden, he has pretty much committed to a life of physical cutoff and emotional distance from all his parents.[217] After so much parenting, the dude needed some space. Once things kick off with Naomi, Holden has a change of heart. He wants his parents to know the new Belter in his life. So Holden begins the complicated but ultimately worthwhile process of renegotiating rules, roles, and boundaries with his eight parents. That's love.

Bowen felt pretty confident that the only way for you to become differentiated was through renegotiations of relationship dynamics with your family of origin. But we gotta disagree with Grandpapa Bowen on this one. For some of us, it just isn't possible to have an IRL renegotiation for all kinds of reasons, not the least of which are personal safety and/or death-related. Jessica Jones certainly has elements of this in her own character evolution—in both the comics and the Netflix series. Before she learns that some of her family of origin might still be kicking, Jessica reckons with the tragic impact of their death and the conflicted relationships she had with them.[218] Eventually, Jessica is able to forgive herself for fighting with her brother and parents before their death because she comes to understand that these dynamics between a teenager, a younger sibling, and overworked parents are normal. This realization not only helps Jessica to make peace with the past but also helps her to shift her stuck dynamics with her friend and surrogate sister[lxxx] from teenage conflict to adult compassion.

If you're a fan of the indie game *Night in the Woods,* you may have anticipated where we're going with this next example.[219] If so, say it with us: Angus the bear! As a cub, Angus was the victim of neglect, physical abuse, and emotional abuse perpetrated by his parents. As an adult, he feels it is

[lxxx] Trish Walker in the Netflix series and Carol Danvers in the comics (*Alias,* vol. 1, #6, 2002).

neither safe nor possible to renegotiate emotional ties with his family of origin. But all is not lost for Angus, prince of bears![lxxxi] As he matures, Angus engages in mindful reflection on his own and with supportive friends. This new chosen family helps him to heal from his past and learn how to make different kinds of emotional connections in the present. You may recall from chapter 7 that we tend to re-create part of the dynamics observed and/or engaged in during early childhood. This tendency can set the stage for some powerful healing, allowing for a corrective emotional experience. Let's take another look at Angus. In the video game, Angus befriends your avatar Mae, a cat struggling with some trauma of her own in addition to some mood-disorder symptoms (think back to the anxiety gremlins and the depression Demogorgon). He is also in a committed romantic partnership with Gregg, a fox with lots of energy and, dare we say, rage issues.[lxxxii] It doesn't take a Jefferson Starship therapist to realize that these new friends and Angus have the potential to play out some old and painful dynamics from Angus's family of origin. But they also have the potential to heal old emotional wounds if Angus and his friends can find new and different ways to interact with one another.

Thank You for Being a Friend

Our families of origin can be less than ideal, and we can still have supportive others in our lives. Enter the chosen family, which is exactly what it sounds like. It's the people we've chosen to shamble around this big rock with, even if we aren't tied by blood familial bond.[220] As Bobby Singer of the *Supernatural* chosen family once said, "Family don't end with blood."[lxxxiii] Innumerable examples of chosen families exist in fandom. It tends to be the strange and outcast who find themselves alone and in need of comfort.

[lxxxi] This is his title in our headcanon because Angus is the sweetest and literal best, i.e., a prince of bears.

[lxxxii] Who doesn't love hitting glass bottles with bats in empty parking lots from time to time, amirite?

[lxxxiii] Have you seen those Jordandené T-shirts? We've got ten of them.

Think the island of misfit toys from the 1964 *Rudolph the Red-Nosed Reindeer*, but with less judgment and clay. Whether one has been rejected, misunderstood, or abandoned by their family, chosen family can stand in where family of origin cannot.

Chosen families have a long history and a special place in the hearts of those in marginalized communities. In times when families of origin rejected their queer relatives, LGBTQIA+ folks had to find a safe chosen family in order to get their needs met. Chosen families were also common for those who moved out of small towns and into the big city, where they had no family. Chosen families provide safety, support, and sharing of resources.

We think that one of the best and most beloved chosen families in the history of television is *The Golden Girls*.[221] For those of you familiar with this fandom, you might be wondering about Dorothy and Sophia. Remembering from chapter 5 offers a helpful explanation: though Sophia has been Dorothy's "ma" all her life, these two adult women renegotiate (or remember) their relationship to one another due to the influence of the community of friends and housemates to which they now belong. By engaging with one another as peers within the context of their new friend and housemate community, the two become chosen family in addition to their familial bond. The golden girls have all been through some tremendous loss and lean on one another to help them through the trials and tribulations of aging in American eighties and early nineties culture. The four often have more diffuse boundaries than flexible—not everybody consented to your sexcapade tirade, Blanche—but when it comes to the hard stuff, they keep it real with straight talk and a slice of cheesecake. Chosen family can be sought out at any time of life, but doing so during transitional periods, such as after a breakup, divorce, or death, is common.

Gargoyles[lxxxiv] is another excellent example of the healing powers of chosen family that can both inspire and foster positive change within our family of origin.[222] After the gargoyles reawaken to find themselves in 1990s New York City, they meet two very different humans: David Xanatos,[lxxxv]

[lxxxiv] The mid-1990s cartoon, not that terrible live-action TV movie from 1972. #werenotcomingforyou

[lxxxv] Voiced by *Star Trek: The Next Generation* heartthrob Jonathan Frakes.

the devilishly handsome Greek zillionaire, and the kind and compassionate biracial Detective Elisa Maza.[lxxxvi] These two relationships mark a turning point for the newly awakened gargoyles. Will they double down on the fear and anger caused by their shared trauma of their rookery brothers being murdered by Vikings in 1200 AD and turn against humanity? Or will they accept the hand of friendship Elisa offers? The gargoyles use flexible boundaries along with the trust staircase and get to know Elisa and Xanatos, ultimately deciding to choose Elisa as family. Her inclusion into the gargoyle family unit helps them to heal from the trauma of another family member's betrayal[lxxxvii] and actualize as individuals: they get names, they learn new skills like how to write computer code, and Goliath and Elisa start a cross-species romance (maybe).

We'll Make Great Pets[lxxxviii]

In addition to our chosen human family, we must always respect the other magical creatures who help us each get through the day. We are of course referring to the animal friends who enrich our lives and our experience of the world; human beings don't have a monopoly on joy and connection. Princess Mononoke of the titular Studio Ghibli film is kinda not into people.[223] To be fair to her, modern human beings have done her and her magical creatures pretty dirty. Plus, she's been raised by magic wolf-gods,[lxxxix] and, with no clear memory of human parents, she takes the animals of the forest as both her family of origin and chosen family. So who could blame her for being more trusting of fur friends? This happens IRL as well. Pets just don't let us down the same way people can. The thing with critters is that they run on emotion. They don't have big plans or ulterior motives, aside from

---

[lxxxvi] Initially envisioned as a Hispanic character, the creators of the cartoon changed Elisa's ethnic background to match that of the voice actress's identities: African American and Indigenous.

[lxxxvii] Yeah, we're talking about you, Demona—voiced by the amazing Marina Sirtis.

[lxxxviii] If you haven't yet, we strongly encourage you to hop on that YouTube and search for this classic early nineties song by the band Porno for Pyros. It's a pun (we think).

[lxxxix] Pretty dope, right?

getting an extra treat. Mostly all they want is to love and be loved. Sure, they might mess up and maybe eat your favorite hat, but you forgive them almost instantly because that's true love.

Animals can help humans learn to love again. Have you ever been to an airport, sat down with a warm beverage, and looked up to see a friendly airport service dog making eyes and wagging its tail at you? How about an airport pony?[xc] Emotional support animals help humans to relax and recenter during stressful situations. They can also be used in therapy to help folks experience unconditional love in a safe space. So when you see a show like *Chilling Adventures of Sabrina*[224]—or read the eponymous comic of the same name[225]—you might want to notice the ways her familiar Salem shows up for her as she does magic. Your beloved tabby cat can fill a similar role in your magical life. Or think of Lyra and her daemon from the *His Dark Materials* book series.[226] Yes, friends, all creatures are magical creatures, and they can be a powerful part of your family of choice.

Let's pause here and take a moment to journal or reflect on your family of choice. Who's in it? Who do you wish was in it? Consider the rules, roles, and boundaries of your family of choice. Without attaching any meaning to what comes up, just notice. Then take some time to reflect on how you feel about this chosen family and your place in it.

[xc] They're real, and they're spectacular.

FANFIC CASE STUDY:
The Expanse, All Together Now

"Welcome aboard the *Roci*," the big man says, waving us forward. We each stumble in our respective space suits, grumbling to one another about whether or not we made the right choice accepting the *Rocinante* crew's invitation to do an intensive family therapy session with them *en vivo*, a therapeutic practice that means engaging the family in their home during a time of peak conflict.

We recall the tight beam transmission from Alex and Amos:

"You won't regret it," Alex Kumal, *Roci*'s pilot and apparently the owner of this particular great idea, assured us.

"Definitely not," his compatriot and the big man in question said, his voice booming and his affect coming through decidedly fast across the tight beam message.

So here we are, pulling ourselves through the airlock and clamping our grav boots down to one of the flat walls that seems to be the floor (at least for now), so as to better extricate ourselves from our space suits.

"Let me help you with that. I'm Amos," says a man who grasps one of our helmets and plucks it off like a child might pop off the head of a daisy.

"Pleasure to meet you, Amos."

"Is it?" Amos asks with a monotone inflection.

We exchange nods and both agree; our initial assessment that Amos may be on the autism spectrum seems to be bearing out. "Yes, we think so. We've heard a lot about you and the *Rocinante*. And only half of them have been negative."

At this, Amos busts into a smile—the first facial expression we've seen from him. "Jokes. I like you two already. Here, lemme get your helmet."

In a matter of seconds, we are free of our space suits and floating among the tools from what looks to be a workshop. We hear the slight *fizztz* of air and look left to see Alex Kumal, live and in person, float toward us.

"Howdy, there, Docs. Helluva a ride up from Brakebills. Y'all feelin' all right? Antigrav meds weren't too hard on you, were they?"

We chuckle. "After the rocket up, it's pretty much been all uphill."

"Jokes," Amos claps us across the backs, "keep 'em comin'. Cap loves jokes right, Alex?"

Alex's brow furrows. "Well he might not like this one."

Alex's compatriot shrugs. "Has to be this way. No other option."

We stare into Amos's face but can't get anything from him. Our gaze shifts to Alex, who does not meet our eyes.

"Well, now's as good a time as any, I expect." Alex blows out a lungful of air and says, "Cap and Naomi, they don't exactly know you're coming."

"They don't know at all," Amos continues. "This is more like a surprise."

"An intervention," Alex corrects.

Amos shifts to hover next to him. "Right, an intervention. Well, best to frame it as a surprise for Cap. Don't think he'll take kindly to an intervention."

"Excuse us, but are we to understand that neither James Holden nor Naomi Nagata know about this family therapy session?"

"Don't worry," comes a voice from the upper deck of the ship. "You're just in time to tell them."

"Cap! And right on time. Should we make coffee for the session?" Amos asks, glancing around at what is fast becoming a cramped workshop. "Hmm, better move to the galley, don't you think?" We pause for a moment, considering if we could ask for tea instead but think better of it, considering we are being hosted and the *Rocinante* crew are decidedly coffee drinkers.

James Holden hovers in front of us, flanked by the infamous Naomi Nagata. Naomi, at least, seems to be having fun—her black eyes sparkle with a smile that hasn't yet made it down to the bottom of her face. Holden, on the other hand, looks to be not the least bit amused, his strong jaw set in a firm "don't mess with Texas" pout. Naomi shoves Holden gently and says, "We might as well hear them out over coffee."

As we make our way to the galley, we notice the tension move through the crew. While Amos's face stays set in a neutral expression to rival the chillest monk, his fingers twitch incessantly—thumbs tapping on the index finger to the middle finger and back to index then to pinky. Alex's feelings are easy to read: his nervous glances and set jaw tell us that he's resolute in the choice he made while totally unsure how this will turn out. Holden holds his feelings close to the spacesuit and might benefit from individual therapy to unravel his childhood rebellion against his communal lifestyle. Also, he's clearly got a raging coffee addiction. Naomi is perhaps the only member of the family who remains somewhat of an emotional mystery to us. But we love a challenge!

Lost in thought, we nearly bump into Amos grabbing the side of the entranceway into the galley. Amos prepares and passes around the coffee bulbs, and we each take a seat.

"So, who's going to explain this?" Holden begins, furrowing his wooly brow at us.

"I can, Cap," Amos volunteers, leaning back in his seat and stretching out his legs. "Things just haven't been right between you and Naomi—hell, you and all of us—since that run-in with Naomi's ex."

"That was certainly a way of putting it," Naomi interrupts, pulling a curl of hair down over her forehead. She sighs into her bulb of coffee. "But Amos is right. We've been off, though I probably would have tracked it back to when you came back up from visiting Earth."

Alex shakes his head. "Nothing good comes from going home."

Holden visibly bristles, shoulders raising almost to his ears. "Well, not all of us abandoned our family, Alex."

"Jim," Naomi's soft voice bends to a lower octave, "that wasn't necessary." Her Belter patois is subtler than we expected. She's clearly been living among this family of choice for a long time.

"I don't see you rushing back home to your polyamory farm commune," Alex shoots back, hunching forward over his bulb.

"My parents aren't all polyamorous," Holden shoots back, showing the whites of his eyes, "they're part of a group marriage. It's common on Mars too."

"Hell, I know that," Alex looks up at his captain, his eyes wet. "But that was a low blow about my kid and ex back on Mars. I know I let them down. I couldn't be the husband or father they needed, and I couldn't face that. So, I ran. But I'm not doin' that now, am I?"

"No, this time you lied about getting us all together for a family therapy session."

"Only because I knew you'd say no and we need help. C'mon, Holden, look around. We all care about you. But this here family is not working the way it used to."

We take a sip of our coffee, and at least one of us is pleased by its depth of flavor. We take a deep breath and reply, "Do each of you consider yourselves a part of this family?"

"Yeah," Amos looks us straight in the eyes. "This is it for me, Docs. These people right here. Been around enough liars and cheats to know real family when I see it."

Naomi smiles at Amos. "And here I thought you were only loyal to me."

Amos turns to her and shrugs. "It ain't been like that for a while now, Naomi. I'm . . . sorry I didn't say anything."

"Thank you, but it's all right, Amos. I knew. And you're right. It is better this way."

"I didn't exactly say that," Amos replies, scratching at his head.

"It seems to be the case for all of you," we interrupt then, inviting the entire crew into the discussion. "This family that you built certainly has traces of the familial groups from which you came. But this family seems to be decidedly different for each of you."

"Hmm, could you say more about that, Doc?" asks Alex, looking a bit confused. "I think I get what you mean, but I'm also kinda not sure."

We smile at Alex. He certainly did some research about family therapy before he sent out the request for us to visit.

"Of course, Alex. Well, for one, it seems like your previous family back on Mars had a lot of secrets—some that you kept from them and, our guess is, some that they kept from you."

"That's true," Alex replies, cocking his head to the side. "My ex did always seem pretty fond of my flight buddy."

"But she never talked to you directly about it?" we ask.

"No," Alex smiles sadly, "we didn't have that kinda relationship."

"And yet it sounds like you want to have that kind of relationship here with your fellow crewmates?"

"Family members," Amos cuts in.

We nod. "You're absolutely right—family members. It sounds like you each want to have the rule of no secrets from each other, at least no secrets around big issues that concern the entire family. You each want honesty, but it's been hard to enact that rule."

"Hmm, sometimes. I think we did pretty good at first, when we were in crisis and on the run from everyone. But since the ring gates opened and after Miller was kickin' around in Cap's head... things haven't felt the same."

"It was me," Naomi says quietly, looking up from the table. "I broke the honesty rule first. I should have told Jim about my son. I should have told all of you."

"I mean, I figured," Amos answers. Alex and Holden turn to stare at him in surprise. Amos shrugs. "She was always so cagey around kids. And remember that time we were celebrating after Avasarala got appointed as head minister of Earthers—"

"Prime minister," Alex corrected.

"Who cares? Anyway, we were all drunk, and Holden asked us how we'd all feel about being uncles if he and Naomi had kids. Naomi got sick, like, immediately afterward. Spent the rest of the night in the head."

"I'm sorry, Amos. I shouldn't have asked you to keep that a secret."

Amos looked down at his hands. "You didn't. I just knew. I can pick up on shit like that. Getting abandoned and pimped out does that to a person."

"Amos, wha?" Alex sputters. "That happened to you when you were a kid?"

"It's not a big deal."

"Perhaps it is a deal," we offer.

Amos turns, "Not a big one."

We hold up our hands to clarify. "But those early experiences of exploitation taught you how to read people and, more specifically, dangerous situations."

"That's true," Amos answers.

"And there's been danger on this ship. And the danger is what happens when a secret is kept so long that it starts to fester."

"Like that proto-molecule goop on the *Roci*'s underbelly that let ghost Miller into Cap's head!" Amos replies.

For a moment we are completely thrown off. But years of training helps us to take these strange revelations in stride. In family therapy, it's far more about the process than the content being shared. "Yes, exactly, Amos. Secrets make us sick."

Holden sighs and shifts in his chair. "This is all my fault."

"No," we say gently, "this is not all about what you did or didn't do here, Jim. This is about all of you coming together now and healing from the pain of secrets."

"OK, well, how do we do it then?"

"Yeah," asks Alex, "how do we heal?"

"It's going to be a process," Naomi answers. "It's not something that can be done all in one day."

"But we only got the Docs for like thirty-six more hours," Amos counters.

"We might be able to stay a bit longer," we reply, "provided that's all right with the captain."

There is a long silence in which each family member looks to Holden. Holden shakes his head, his shoulders easing back down as Naomi slips a hand under his arm. "Well, it's like you said, Docs. It's not up to me. It's up to all of us. We're not just a scrappy bunch of survivors anymore. We're a family. And yeah, we've all kept things from each other, shoved it under the bulkhead because we thought saying it out loud would push the others away. But it's the hiding that's done the pushing. So I'm in this if all of you are. If the Docs can stay for a while, I'm with all of you. Let's heal this family. It's the most important thing to me, across all the galaxies behind each of those ring gates."

Naomi squeezes his arm. "It's the most important thing to me, too, Jim."

Alex grins so wide it looks like he might bust. "You know I'm here."

"Shit. Bunch of babies," Amos smiles. "I'd kill anyone for you three."

Alex hugs Amos. And though the big man at first looks like he might choke the smaller one, he reluctantly hugs him back.

"Group hug!" Holden shouts.

We smile to ourselves. This family is getting it back together.

FANFIC CASE STUDY QUESTIONS:
Put on Your Spacesuit and Consider the Following!

- How do each of the crew's families of origin impact the way they initially connect with their fellow crew members?
- What is the turning point in the session when they realize that they are more than "just a scrappy bunch of survivors"?
- Now think about your own family of origin. What are some struggles that you currently face that are similar to those of your parents? Your grandparents?
- Consider your chosen family. In what ways does this chosen family both mirror and counter patterns in your family when you were growing up?

THE EXPANSE MEDITATION:

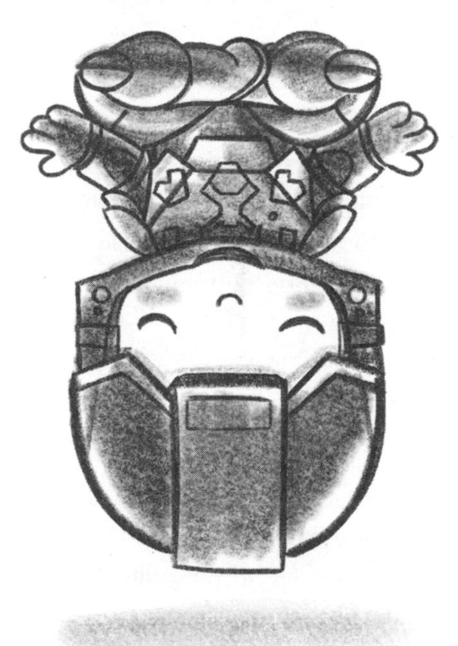

The following meditation is meant to help you to get the emotional feeling of boundaried space between yourself and those around you. If we are going to go into space, or, rather, into the greater space that we share with others, we must affix our spacesuit to ensure our own safety. This meditation is useful any day but especially so when you will interact with people or in places that you know test your boundaries. Once you've done this meditation, you can always simply remember your space suit and conjure it up quickly in the moment.

Find a comfortable seat or place to lie down. Take a moment to pause and take a few deep, cleansing breaths. Considering going out into space can be daunting. As you rest, begin to focus on your breathing. There's no need to control your breathing; just notice what the air feels like as it comes in and goes out. Once you feel that your mind and body are in a state of calm, or as close to calm as is possible today, imagine that you are standing on a spaceship. You've been called on a mission where you will need to don your spacesuit for your protection.

Take a moment to notice what the spacesuit looks like, and when you're ready, start to put it on.

Starting with the main body of the suit, picture that it fits firmly around your body but is not constricting.

Next, step into your boots, and affix them to the body of your suit. Pay attention to the connections—the straps, the ties, and the tassels—and make sure they are secure.

Then put on your gloves, making sure that they are affixed securely. You may want to flex each hand once it is in place to ensure that you can move your fingers in them.

Pause and take a breath before putting on your helmet. It can be a bit scary to think about relying on your suit to supply your oxygen. Just remember that this is what the suit was built for. It was made to protect you, and its entire job is to keep you safe.

Once you feel ready, put on your helmet. Turn it left and then turn it right to lock it into place. Notice how it feels to be fully enveloped in the safe confines of your space suit.

Before you embark on your journey, take a few more moments to breathe as you check each of the fasteners on your space suit. Make sure that all your connections are secure so that you can maintain this wonderful oxygen you have flowing through your system. Any loose edges could cause dangerous space to seep into your suit and suck out your air. Once your suit feels fully secure, make your way to the door of your space station.

Take a few more deep breaths, and return to the real world with the image of your space suit fully intact, so that as you exit out into the space of the real world you feel just as secure as you did inside your own mind.

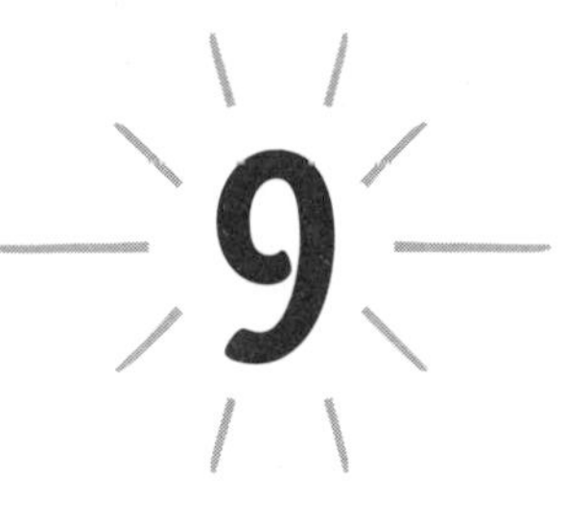

Are Video Games the Big Bad?

It's so much easier to measure life in experience points.

—**CODEX, *THE GUILD***[227]

Every time something new is invented, folks think of how it is going to be the ruin of us all. Whether it was the printed word, the telephone, or the television, a group of cranks shouted, "Not on my lawn." The irony, of course, is that these inventions ultimately brought the human race closer together emotionally, rather than driving it apart. Since their inception, video games have been maligned as sheer escapism. Once violence and sex were introduced in games, they became the scapegoats for any correlation between a gamer and violence. Remember, friends, correlation does not equal causation.

Correlate Your Cause

Imagine you're on the bridge of the Starship Enterprise with Kirk and Spock. You just got a new ensign pip on your collar, and you're feeling dapper. Just as you're about to approach the captain, the bridge doors slide open, and Uhura strides onto the bridge with her afternoon cup of coffee.[xci] You turn to look and trip over the bridge railing, landing into one James T. Kirk's lap. How embarrassing! Or, maybe, thrilling? Probably both. Now, did Uhura's entrance onto the bridge cause you to trip over the railing? No. Unfortunately, you're just clumsy. But because these two instances happened simultaneously, an outside observer might read connection, or *causation,* into these events, when, in fact, the only thing going on here is *correlation* and a lack of gross motor control. Now, if Uhura strides onto the bridge and throws her coffee at you because she doesn't like your smug new-pip-having face and then you fall over the railing, Uhura is the cause of your fall. That's causation. Notice the difference.

The psychological research done on violent video games suggests only a correlation between violent gaming and violent action, not causation.[228] The nuance in both the research and the ongoing debate of the impact of video games lies in our feelings. Just like movies, television, and books, video games impact our emotions. This makes a lot of sense when we recall what we learned back in chapter 3: emotions give us messages about our relationship with our internal reality as well as information about our external environment. So a video game can cause us to feel mad or sad or smad. But video games have never been shown to cause an individual to attack someone with a coffee mug—regardless of whether that someone was being real smug about their new pips.

What happens if video games tap into our emotions, getting us all riled up with feelings of smadness? Well, video games offer us an opportunity to discharge these feelings.[229] And by that we mean they offer the opportunity for healthy coping skills.[230] Remember the shadow tools that we discussed in chapter 6? Many folks view video games in the same shadow category as alcohol and overmuch pie, and, sure, folks can overdo it in the world of gaming, too (more on that in a bit). But at its core, there is nothing inherently shadowy about playing video games. Gaming allows us to activate uncomfortable feelings and engage with them in a safe space. They also offer the opportunity for catharsis, or the ability to release anger in a safe way.

[xci] Yes, we know caffeine can be problematic for some, but Uhura knows what she's doing.

If video games provide emotional catharsis—and they definitely do[231]—then they might have some self-care properties. Let's pause for a moment. Have any thoughts or feelings come up for you as we've begun to question the social norms around video gaming? Perhaps video games have been important to you for a long time, and memories of receiving negativity or critical judgment around gaming are coming up for you. Or maybe you've never played a video game in your life, and this all seems a little strange and maybe even far-fetched. Perhaps you're wondering, *How could a first-person shooter be even remotely cathartic?* All thoughts and questions are welcome. Without assigning any judgment to what comes up, just notice your feelings. If it feels helpful, you might want to write down some of these feelings either in your journal or in the journal of your mind palace.

The Gates of Hell

Problem gaming isn't the only problem in games. If you are a gamer, then you probably already know where we are going with this: Gamergate. In 2014, a group of gamers took to the internet to troll two gaming-industry figures, Zoë Quinn and Brianna Wu, and the lone woman at the time critiquing games, Anita Sarkeesian. The trolling wasn't the fun-under-the-bridge kind; it was more of the break-your-bones-and-traumatize-your-mind kind.[232] Though the argument has been made that violent video games rife with sexist and racist stereotypes caused Gamergate, we offer that—rather than video games causing harm—fear of change, mob mentality, and social capital were the main driving forces. The time of Gamergate was terrible for the gaming subculture, frightening people out of the industry, pushing people offline, and severely altering many lives. However, there are reasons to be hopeful that the industry itself has started to engage in some posttraumatic growth. Representation within games has expanded significantly, leading to more inclusive and diverse storylines and characters.[233] Gaming companies made some progress in diversity initiatives, though there is still a long way to go when it comes to consistently hiring women, men, and gender-nonbinary people from a wide variety of racial and ethnic backgrounds. Though much work still remains to be done, the gaming industry and surrounding community as a whole has generally leveled up its awareness.

Gamergate continues to serve as a call to action to be mindful of the makers of our games, their stories and characters, and the folks with whom we play. It invites us all to critically engage with the Westworld Constructs that were once norms of the gaming industry and to co-create a new gaming construct where we can all win. Loving a gaming franchise does not prohibit the ability to think critically about its flaws. For example, we genuinely love *The Legend of Zelda* series even as we readily admit its problematic elements.

If you engage in online gaming, then you've probably encountered a troll or ten. If you do encounter a troll, remember your communication skills and self-care. Assume neutral intent and get curious while regularly checking in with your own self-care needs. If trolls show that they have negative intent, then you get to do what is best for you, whether that means logging off or asking them to leave your team.

Level Up Your Self-Care

Later on, we'll address the drops in the room related to gaming addiction.[xcii] For now, let's use the Westworld Construct to question the accepted norms that video games negatively impact the lives of gamers. What if video games were like a hammer[xciii]—a neutral tool that could be used in a variety of ways, resulting in a variety of outcomes depending on the way it is used? Remember when we talked about the cathartic relief of defeating your gaming opponents? That applies to all kinds of feelings, and such catharsis can actually lead to healing when paired with tools of Therapeutic Fanfiction.

If you're a gamer, you may want to think about the games and characters that help you make sense of what's going on in your own life. If, for instance, you have difficulties in decision-making, then perhaps the game *Undertale* could help you play out what different choices might look like. In

[xcii] *Drops* refers to the special gifts left in a combat area that a player's video game avatar can pick up and use after defeating the big bads.

[xciii] A hammer used to gently hit a nail into a wall to hang a portrait is so helpful! A hammer used to hammer a nail into your roommate's television because they will not stop watching *Love Island* is destructive.

this game, you have the option to never fight anyone. You can be kind the entire time, and that results in different outcomes, just like in the real world! However, just like in the real world, your kindness is not always met with kindness. Interactions with other beings—monsters and humans alike—are not bidirectional cause-and-effect loops. Your decision to be kind will not guarantee a specific or desired response in any of the many ghosties you encounter in *Undertale* or in everyday life.

Another example of a video game that pairs well with Therapeutic Fanfiction is *Celeste*. If you're familiar with this game, you're probably already thinking of Celeste Mountain and just how long it took you to climb certain parts of it. One of us in particular got to a point in the game where she truly believed that she would never make it out of Mr. Oshiro's haunted hotel.[xciv] But if you can use the tool of externalization, you can see that the challenging aspects of *Celeste* re-create the challenge of change. Behavior change of any kind takes a long time. Do you remember learning to walk? On second thought, you probably don't. But have you ever seen babies learning to walk? They fall down a billion times. They get bruises. They cry. Hell, even learning to crawl usually takes months. The idea that change should be fast or easy is totally incorrect. The Therapeutic Fanfiction tools of Westworld Construct, externalization, and fandom attachment can help you learn and integrate this truth all while video gaming. Bringing this awareness to *Celeste* can help to normalize not just gaming difficulty but also the difficulty inherent in everything you might be trying to change in your daily life.

Ch-ch-ch-changes

Now is as good a time as any to talk about the transtheoretical model of change, aka PCP in the AM.[234] This is a fun mnemonic for remembering the stages of change: precontemplation, contemplation, preparation, action, and maintenance. Precontemplation is exactly what it sounds like. You haven't considered making a change yet. Maybe someone has said

[xciv] That red mold meant business.

to you that they think you could stand to change something. But you're like, "Nah, I'm good." The shift from precontemplation to contemplation happens over time. Perhaps enough people have commented on a need for change, or you've started noticing that things aren't going quite how you'd like them to. Contemplation requires a lot of reflection and conversation with trusted community. In the preparation stage, you start to gather resources. You consider different options and choose one that you think would be the best. This is also known as the research phase of change. Notice all the steps that need to happen before the action stage. Change is slow.

And now you move into action. You do the thing you said you were gonna do. Change leads organically into the final stage of the model, maintenance. During this phase, you repeat the new behavior change numerous times until it becomes a pattern and then eventually a habit. During maintenance, another phase can occur: regression or relapse. Both of these words carry with them a heavy dose of shame and guilt. But falling back into old shadow tools can be a helpful part of the change process. Regression gives you the chance to experience an old tool in a new way because though the tool is the same, you are different. You get the opportunity to see how different it feels and decide whether this tool serves you. It's a reminder of why you made changes in the first place. While you can certainly apply this model to any video game of your choice, we're going to apply it to video gaming in general. Let's break it down:

1. Precontemplation: You've been hearing about that new game on the interwebs. Peeps have been talking about it all over Discord, and you're intrigued.
2. Contemplation: While talking with your gamer pals, you bring up said game and ask if they know it. A close pal says yes and that they loved it! You think, *Hey, maybe I should check out this game.*
3. Preparation: You decide to get serious and look up this game on Steam.[xcv] Damn! It's more money than you wanted to spend. So now you shift back up to the contemplation stage and think about it

[xcv] A digital storefront and social service for games. We promise, it's fun.

some more. After some really solid reflection and a few more friends saying how much they love said game, you decide to take the plunge! Of course, you need to wait for it to download. And, while you wait, you probably purchase some gaming fuel—pizza, soda, and snacks. Or maybe kale chips. We're not here to judge.

4. Action: The time is now! You open that game and start to play but then—the dreaded tutorial level.[xcvi] As you continue to play the video game, you'll learn all sorts of new in-game tricks and techniques, which means that you'll cycle through this change model numerous times as you play. If you're playing a temple-based game, like one of the myriad *Zelda* games, you'll no doubt recall that each temple, or level, gets progressively harder, ideally to match and then challenge your new skill level. This is where gaming and IRL change mimic each other: you sometimes think that you're regressing or backsliding when in fact you've just gotten more skills and have taken on a new more challenging quest.
5. Maintenance: At this point, you're a pro at this game. If it's open world, then you've seen a lot of shit and battled a lot of big bads. Now, you can pretty much roam: go where you wanna go and do what you wanna do for hours without risking an in-game death.

Video-Gaming Your Self-Care

Video games, much like Doctor Who's TARDIS, are bigger on the inside. Games are important because they help us engage with our possibly neglected and ignored inner child. They encourage play, foster creativity, and encourage community-building. We've included the following brief set of lists to help guide you as you seek out video games that target specific aspects of your own personal self-care. And, if you feel like we've missed a game or ten, add them!

[xcvi] Ugh. Here the game basically tries to explain to you all the bells, whistles, and tricks for how to play. But you're going to learn all that as you go along. Plus, that's what the internet is for.

Distraction

Fortnite: That game that Drake loves. It's a co-op shooter game that lets you outfit your avatar with nifty gear and skins (i.e., different costumes). It's kinda like *Animal Crossing* but with guns.

Call of Duty: Shoot people, but don't be a dick. Just because you're shooting people in co-op gaming mode does not mean you need to use violent racist language.

Minecraft: Build shit with blocks!

Candy Crush Saga: But, really, any and all phone games apply here. Gaming—it's not just for the television.

Healing

Journey: Get ready to weep while you play the archetypal hero's journey.

Night in the Woods: Because who doesn't love anthropomorphic cats who engage in crimes?

Celeste and *Hyper Light Drifter*: Explore complicated topics like differentiation and the transtheoretical model of change via the joys of dungeon crawling and mountain climbing.

Mindfulness

Stardew Valley: Chill out. Plant some kale. Flirt with some grocery-store clerks. Honestly, what more could you ask for?

Monument Valley: A game of puzzles and suspense!

Flower: A beautiful and soothing game that answers the question "what if you were a flower?"

Animal Crossing: New Horizons: It's like *Fortnite* but without guns. On your own personal island, you get to design everything right down to your cupola and dancing shoes.

Highway to the Shadow Zone

Whereas our bias is that gaming is a healthy coping skill, we cannot deny that, just like anything else in this life, your use of it can become harmful. A helpful place to start is to consider the amount of time you spend gaming relative to other aspects of your life. You may want to consider some or all of the following: the quality of your sleep, meaning-making activities, your relationship with food, and body movement.

Does it serve you to stay up until 4:00 a.m. gaming when you have to work at 7:00 a.m.? Well, it was probably fun during the gaming portion but really hard during the morning-after portion. Perhaps it would better serve you to head to bed around 2:00 a.m. We're not going to tell you to go to bed at 10:00 p.m. and shut off all your screens thirty minutes before you lie down. We're not monsters. However, if a therapist has recommended this to you in the past, they aren't monsters either (probably)—they just don't understand gaming culture. All gaming devices that involve screens expose you to increased amounts of artificial blue light. Prolonged blue-light exposure can lead to eye strain, disordered sleep, and migraines.

When pondering meaningful activities, you may want to consider the amount of time you spend engaging with other human beings. Gaming with other humans counts, but we want to make sure that we have both kinds of relationships: virtual and IRL. One of the most common misconceptions that plague folks inside and outside of therapy is "IRL bias," or bias for friendships out in the "real world" as opposed to online friendships via chat, Zoom, text, or online games. Now, this isn't to say that virtual hangs should replace IRL hangs or vice versa. What we're offering is that both are real forms of human interaction and connection. It's really more about what is speaking to you right now and what you presently have access to rather than an either-or, one-size-fits-all approach.

Both movement and food carry a lot of cultural baggage. The key is to remember that you get to choose what baggage to keep and what baggage to pass back. Again, we must discuss the importance of balance. In our clinical practices, we talk a lot about a style of eating called attuned eating.

The idea is to pay attention to your body's cues related to hunger, energy, and satiation or fullness. We often describe this process as a decision tree or a series of nonjudgmental questions that you ask yourself to help identify and parse out emotional, energetic, and nutritional needs.[235] Gaming can cause you to lose track of time, which means that you aren't thinking about meals. Nor are you tuned in to internal cues telling you to take a break and eat. Gamers will sit down with a bag of snacks to munch on during play, which might not provide the type of energy your body needs. We invite you to take breaks while you're playing, to move your body, use the bathroom, and check in on your physical hunger. You might discover you want to have a snack or even a meal.

Video games and body movement don't need to be mutually exclusive. Think about how fast you punch those keys and twist that joystick when you're in the middle of a boss battle. It's about exploring what's working and when. Your fingers probably need a break from time to time from all that fine motor movement. But before you get up to stretch, let's explore movement.

As you think about the place movement has in your life, consider all types of movement:[xcvii] walking, standing, dancing, sleeping, sitting, running, stretching, Zumba, tap dancing, roller skating, mountain climbing, etc. Before you consider what you might want to change, it can be very helpful to make a list of the ways you already move your body on a regular basis. Because American culture tends to highlight the extremes, many of us have learned to minimize or just ignore many of the ways we move each day. Movement isn't just about how many times you went to the gym, though that could be a component of it. Once you've listed out all the ways you move your body regularly, take a minute to reflect on what movement you tend to really enjoy. As you're doing so, you may realize, for example, that you love walking but don't do it as often as you'd like. Now, you can start to play with ways to increase certain movements (or minimize others). If you look at your list and think, *Wow, none of this sparks joy*, that's OK. This is just information.

Now you have the opportunity for a little experimentation. Consider some movements you haven't tried. If you're having trouble thinking of some,

---

[xcvii] Just like Kenny Powers, we're not asking you to be the best at exercising.

write an *A* to *Z* list, coming up with one movement for each letter. Then try them out. It's unlikely that you will dislike every single one of them. If you find that you do really seem to dislike all of them, that's an opportunity for reflection. What is it that doesn't resonate for you regarding movement? It's possible that your dislike is less about the movements themselves and more about your feelings toward them. You may be trying to make your body fit the movements rather than changing the movements to fit your body. There are ways to adapt movements to make them more accessible. Sadly, not all fitness instructors understand this practice. When you learn new movements from an instructor (on the internet, a book, or IRL), they might instruct in a way that doesn't work for you. Use the Westworld Construct tool to ask if you can change the movements to be more authentic to you.

We invite you to be mindful of the balance in your own life with compassion. We are never completely in harmony; the goal is to not get too out of tune. Video games aren't an enemy. They're a tool, just like all the other tools we have in our proverbial tool belt. The challenge is finding a balance to all the aspects of our lives, rather than allowing one to take over. We can engage with video games and have a healthy life. The two are not mutually exclusive.

FANFIC CASE STUDY:
Thomas Was Alone, *Night in the Woods*, *Fortnite*, and *Minecraft*; Welcome to Group

After our time in space, we felt ready to come back to Earth, sort of. To ease our integration, we decide to work virtually via the group therapy model with four current gamer clients: Claire, the big blue superhero cube from *Thomas Was Alone*; Mae, the lovable and sassy anthropomorphic cat from *Night in the Woods*; KingBoss101, the avatar of a player from *Fortnite*; and Kevin from *Minecraft*. The topic of the group focuses on "Processing Emotions." Having gently but firmly explained to KingBoss101 that, no, we could not conduct therapy in the battle arena as a squad, we were ready to begin, but KingBoss101 was not. After brief review of the HIPAA compliance issues, KingBoss101 seemed to understand, or at least to give in for now.

Because this therapy is virtual, we cannot offer our group members tea or other complimentary refreshments. So instead, we offer a piñata shaped like a llama to each member via an email link, which they can use either in *Fortnite* or in the comfort of their gaming environs of choice. Due to the already complicated nature of this therapeutic format, we elect to conduct the group via chat. We log in as <StarshipTherapise1&2> Let the games begin!

—

StarshipTherapise1&2: Welcome to today's group. We're very excited to get to know each of you!

KingBoss101: when do we shoot?

Claire: I was told there would be no violence!

Mae: Crimes! j/k lol

Kevin: Hi, I'm Kevin

StarshipTherapise1&2: As we reviewed in the paperwork, there will be no gaming together for the first 4 weeks of group. This gives us all time to get to know one another and work on communication before moving into more stressful situations.

KingBoss101: i work best under pressure

StarshipTherapise1&2: Well, this is a different sort of pressure. How about we start by going around and saying a little bit about what led you to this group? We already know a bit about each of you, but it would be helpful for you to get to know your group members better.

Kevin: I'll start! I like building things. Like a lot.

Mae: Duh Kevin. You're from Minecraft

Kevin: Why are you mocking me?

Mae: Figure it out

Kevin: Anyways, I'm here because I um I do like building things but it's a lot of alone time. I want to take a pause from building blocks and start to build some friendships

Mae: lame also teacher's pet much?

Kevin: This isn't school. This is group therapy

StarshipTherapise1&2: Kevin, could you tell Mae what it felt like when she teased you?

Mae: *sigh* some peeps just can't take a joke amirite

Kevin: It hurt my feelings. It made me feel like you were saying I'm stupid

Mae: If I thought you were stupid, I'd just tell you to your virtual face, Kevin

StarshipTherapise1&2: Thank you for sharing that, Kevin. It sounds like honesty is important to you, Mae

Mae: idk?!

KingBoss101: is this seriously what we're doing here? talking about feelings?

StarshipTherapise1&2: Pretty much. It's right there in the topic of the group.

Claire: You know, actually, I might be in the wrong group. Yeah, um, I think the email said 0800

Mae: We all got the same email, Claire. I don't like myself either but I'm stuck with me and so are you at least for the next 45 minutes

Kevin: I like you, Mae

StarshipTherapise1&2: Let's pause for a moment. It makes sense that you're all experiencing some big feelings as group is getting started. How about we all take a breath together and return to where we were? Talking about what drew us to this group, which you did want to join, Claire. You've been pretty quiet, why don't you tell us a bit about why you're here?

Claire: I'm here because all my friends are dead

KingBoss101: respawn can be brutal

Claire: My friends and I worked together to save the mainframe but we lost our virtual independence in the process. The lead coder said they'd all come back online eventually. But I'm the first one who has and that was weeks ago. I'm starting to think they might just never come back

KingBoss101: hey Claire man i'm sorry that legit sounds hard one time i got separated from my squad in the middle of a major mission and i just couldn't get back to em ended up just fighting my way through blind but you know what the worst part was

Mae: Is that a question?

Claire: What was the worst part KingBoss101?

KingBoss101: being all alone

Kevin: It sounds like you felt scared and sad KingBoss101

KingBoss101: i was

StarshipTherapise1&2: Thank you so much for sharing that experience, Claire. It sounds like KingBoss101 could really relate to that experience. It seems like we're starting to find some common ground. Mae, where are you at right now?

Mae: uh, my bedroom?

StarshipTherapise1&2: We mean emotionally. What are you *feeling* right now?

Mae: Ugh! I'm feeling...

KingBoss101: scared

Mae: I 100% am not scared KingBoss101

KingBoss101: im not even trying to be mean right now mae

Kevin: Mae, I don't think you are meaning to, but I think you are hurting KingBoss101's feelings

KingBoss101: uhhh i did not say that

Kevin: It can be hard to sit with your feelings. Sometimes, when I'm having a big feeling and I don't know what it is, I go out to the train tracks

Mae: holy shit that's dark

Kevin: No I like to go out there when it's really sunny and then just build some more railroad tracks. There's something about laying down a fresh line of track and then getting in your train car and just watching the scenery slowly roll past you

Mae: Sometimes I feel like that when I go out walking in the woods. Or I did. Now I just feel weird

Claire: Why is that?

Mae: My friends and I kinda killed someone . . . er, like a few people in the woods last year

KingBoss101: howd you do it?

Claire: That sounds really hard

Mae: It was like this weird old god or something. And like a quarter of our town. My friends and I tried to get them out of this weird old hole underground but they were pretty attached to this old god. Plus they were sacrificing other kids in our town to it

KingBoss101: holy fuck dude mae i don't say this lightly i say nothing lightly that may be the most bad-ass thing i have ever heard

Mae: Seriously?

KingBoss101: yeah srsly ive only ever offed husks never a fucking G-O-D!

StarshipTherapise1&2: Mae, it seems like it means a lot to you to hear that KingBoss101 respects you

Mae: I don't care

StarshipTherapise1&2: Well, it seems like you really started to let your guard down when he told you that he's impressed with you

Mae: ugh, I guess. Can we move on?

StarshipTherapise1&2: In a minute. So Mae, you said that you "killed" the god, but if we remember your story right, you were under attack by the god and their followers. You saved the lives of your friends. You all saved each other. I wonder if you could let that narrative in and hold some space instead of letting the "killing" hold all the space?

Claire: I think I kinda know where you're coming from, Mae

Mae: yeah?

Claire: When my friends and I were running from the virus, I helped them all by letting them jump on my back

KingBoss101: fuckin sweet

Claire: There was all this water coming in but see I float in water. I carried all my friends to safety. But I didn't think of myself as having saved them. All I could feel was scared and like overwhelmed

Mae: Yeah because you'd almost died

KingBoss101: yeah but you didnt you made it

Kevin: You are both superheroes

KingBoss101: what kevin said

StarshipTherapise1&2: those were some lovely affirmations. You have all done a great job of sharing a little bit about yourselves and allowing yourselves to have compassion for the others in the group. Great work! Next week we will discuss how to use anger constructively during boss battles

KingBoss101: fuck yeah

Kevin: That could be helpful in defeating the Ender dragon. Tho death brings up complicated feelings for me

Mae: We're here for you kev

Kevin: Thank you, Mae. I'm glad you're here

Claire: I'm glad to be here, too

KingBoss101: me 4 mutherfuckers

StarshipTherapise1&2: Thank you all for *being here* for our first group. You each took risks today in being a little more open with yourselves and with each other. It is through vulnerability that we form our strongest bonds.

FANFIC CASE STUDY QUESTIONS:
Answer Questions, Get XP!

- Which of the four characters did you resonate with most? List a few reasons why they resonated with you. If you connected with all or none, take a few sentences and reflect on what helped you feel either connected or distant from all four.
- At the end of group, StarshipTherapise1&2 offer the reflection that we form our strongest bonds via vulnerability. What feeling came up for you when you read that? Take a moment to reflect without judgment. Once you've written down your feeling, sit with it, and see if that feeling remains or starts to shift.
- What are some of the negative impacts that gaming had on the four group members?
- What are some of the positive impacts that gaming had on the four group members?

YOGA FOR CENTERING:
"I Am a Hero," A Yoga Practice for Calming the Mind and Body Before the Big Boss Battle

The purpose of this yoga practice is to help you get calm and ready for the big boss battle. If you choose to use this yoga practice during game play, pause the game for a moment. Remember that your body is your instrument, and respect its gaming parameters.

1. Seated or Standing Mountain Pose: Find a comfortable stance or sit with your feet firmly on the floor. Notice the feel of your feet on the floor and, if you're seated in a chair, the feel of your body supported by your chair. If it's comfortable, close your eyes. If you'd prefer to keep your eyes open, find something on which to fix your gaze. Start to bring your awareness to your breath. There's no need to control your breathing; just notice what the air feels like as it comes in and goes out.

   Once you start to feel a bit calmer, picture in your mind's eye the *you* in your game. Picture yourself just about to fight the big boss. Notice the feelings as they start to rise in your body.

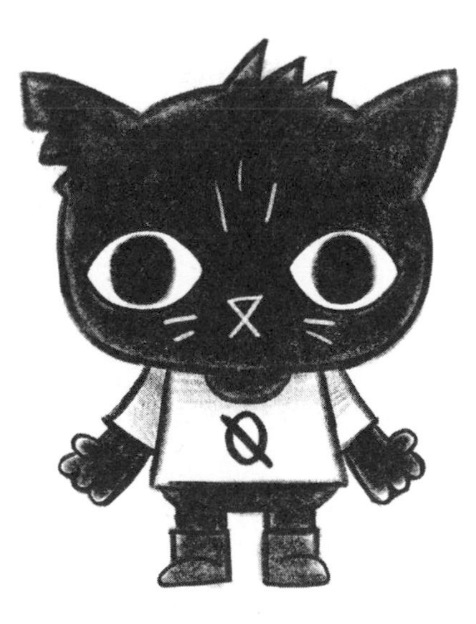

2. Backbend Pose: As the feelings rise up, lift your arms up to the sky. Picture yourself having just defeated your foe. Celebrate this accomplishment by taking a baby backbend and sending out a thank you from your heart. Bring your arms back upward and then down to your heart.

   Allow your awareness to shift to memory. Begin to call upon memories of other times that you have fought virtual or real-life boss battles and won. How did it feel to have succeeded in your quest? Hold on to that feeling, and breathe into it. Allow that feeling to encompass you like a protective shield.

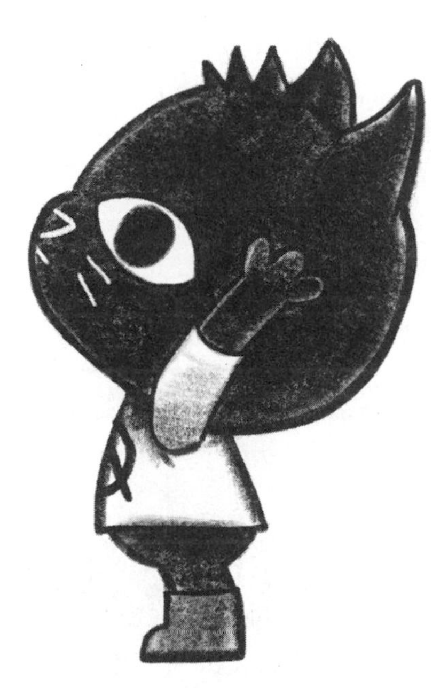

3. Side Stretch Pose: Again, imagine yourself in your game, now with your protective shield fighting your big boss battle. Notice how this feels to you. Sweep your arms up overhead and interlace your fingers, releasing your pointer finger. Explore the edges of your protective shield by moving from right to left, back and forward a few times. If interlacing your fingers is uncomfortable for any reason, keep your arms wide.

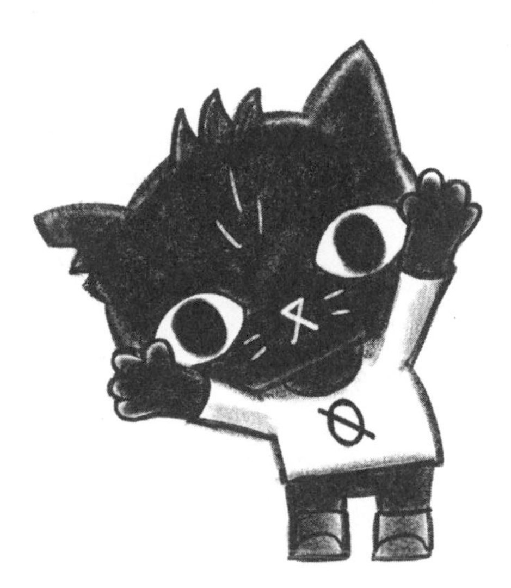

4. Crescent Lunge Pose: Now step one foot forward. You can stay here if that's comfortable, or you can bend your front knee and come up onto the ball mount of your back foot. You can also drop to your back knee. Picture yourself striding to victory. If it helps, you can even move your arms as if you are walking toward your destiny. Hold for five to ten breaths, and then switch sides. Get ready to win.

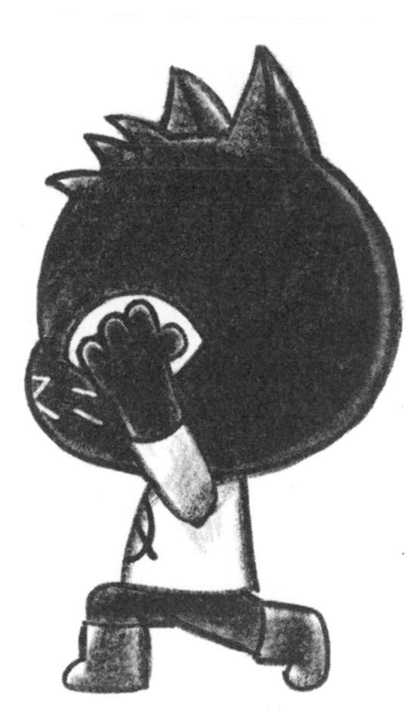

5. Seated or Standing Mountain Pose: Return to your starting pose, and bring your awareness back to your breath. With each inhale, think, *I am,* and with each exhale, *a hero.* Remember this mantra for when you return to the game or any big boss battles that you face.

When It's Time to Find Your Jedi Master, Professor, or Sensei

Therapists are heroic. They're the heroes of listening.

—ZACH GALIFIANAKIS, AS RAY HUESTON IN *BORED TO DEATH*, "STOCKHOLM SYNDROME"[236]

As the two card-carrying members of Starship Therapise, we have a bias: we're very pro-therapy. Pretty much since its inception, therapy has had some critical judgments thrown at it. Some of these were valid: Freud really did have a drug problem, and we're sure that did impact his clinical work. Some of these were not so valid: you only need couples therapy if your partnership is falling apart. And fandom hasn't done the field any favors in its representation of us overall. Therapist John Stamos in *You,* anyone?[xcviii] So, of course, folks are reticent about seeking out therapy. But our rep isn't always bad. There are some amazing therapists in fandom . . . well, one . . . Counselor Deanna Troi.

On *Star Trek: The Next Generation*'s Enterprise, Counselor Troi is part of the bridge crew, meaning that in the future not only is therapy normalized,

---

[xcviii] Therapist John Stamos smokes weed in session, sleeps with his patients, and can't even correctly diagnosis antisocial personality disorder (Siega, et al., 2018–present).

it's also seen as a vital part of Starfleet. The stigma around taking care of your mental health is over, even if Captain Picard has a hard time asking for therapeutic help (he has a hard time asking for help in general). Counselor Troi uses Betazoid empath skills and her Starfleet training to help provide emotional insight into engagements with new species, and she also helps the crew maintain their own mental health. We aren't the only ones who view therapy as important; so did Gene Roddenberry, and we hope you will too.

Let's Talk about Therapy

While we very much hope that this book is helpful to you, it is not meant to replace seeing your own therapist.[xcix] You may already have one, or maybe you've worked with one in the past. Or perhaps you haven't quite been sure when is the "right" time to pursue support from a professional Jedi Master. We hope that wherever you are on this spectrum you're able to find worthwhile information in this chapter. We will touch on all phases of the therapeutic process: researching therapists, reaching out to prospective therapists, setting expectation in therapy, and getting your needs met by your therapist over time.

It can be intimidating looking for a therapist because of the ways helpers tend to be portrayed in fandom. Sometimes the helpers hurt more than they heal. This is one way that the real world differs greatly from our fandoms (hopefully). Let's consider some of the more famous therapeutic fandom figures: Yoda, Gandalf, Professor X. Sometimes these helpers are genuinely helpful. But Yoda is pretty mercurial and also fairly reluctant to take on Luke as a padawan in the first place. And although Gandalf serves as a wise and reassuring presence to his Hobbit friends, he does have an unfortunate habit of abandoning them periodically. Helm's Deep, anyone?[237] Perhaps the most obviously problematic guide is Professor X, who has a habit of manipulating his faithful team[238] and scrambling his X-Men's memories and mutant powers[239] without checking for consent.[c] The main thing that

---

[xcix] For those of you familiar with our podcast, this likely comes as no surprise.

[c] Professor knows best . . . Or does he?

each of these therapeutic figures have in common is that they have a stake in the outcome of their charge's journey. An actual therapist's job is to care for you more than the outcome of the quest. You are not collateral damage to a successful quest.

Let's pause for a moment and consider how you feel about therapy and therapists, both IRL and in fandom. Ponder this without censoring yourself. We'll circle back at the end. For now, we invite you to reflect and record your initial thoughts, musings, assumptions, and/or judgments about therapy.

When Is It Time to Find a Therapist?

The short answer is that there's really never a wrong time to find a therapist. It's a misconception that something specifically needs to be going wrong in your life before you consider therapy. A therapist's entire job is to listen to you and to offer affirmations and support, while offering the occasional (or not so occasional) challenge. Where else in your life is there another human who is there just for you? Friends and family are wonderful, and they also have bias. It's not ill-intentioned, but it's there. For example, way back during the original comic-book run of the *X-Men*, Jean Grey, aka Marvel Girl, wanted to take a break from Scott and the X-Men to explore who she was as an independent person.[240] Neither Scott nor Professor X were great allies for Jean because they had a personal interest in having her stay: Scott wanted his main girl by his side, and Professor X wanted the world's most powerful telekinetic on his team fighting for justice. If Jean had a trusted therapist with super listening powers, they might have been able to validate and normalize her desire to self-actualize. But even on an average day, Jean deals with so much: her growing telepathic abilities, Scott's angst, and mentoring new mutants. Any day would be a good day for her to reach out, and the same goes for you.

We realize that this isn't how everybody feels. And most folks don't have the resources to just be in therapy forever, so folks need to do a bit of discernment. Generally speaking, the time when a therapist will be especially beneficial is when you are experiencing distress that feels overwhelming. Distress can look different and be very subjective. Sometimes folks get bogged down in worrying about what other people will think and are concerned about whether they need or deserve therapy when other people are "doing worse" than they are. Think Bilbo Baggins, who couldn't quite figure out what was bothering him until Gandalf came along and invited him on an adventure.[241] Gandalf sensed his distress and offered support. But in daily life, the helper or therapist won't just appear with a team of Dwarves. You need to reach out, and it doesn't matter if other people get it or not. Do you feel distressed? Does it feel overwhelming? Well, then it doesn't really matter what it looks like to anybody else. Feeling distressed and overwhelmed are reasons enough to reach out to a therapist.

There are more objective ways to tell whether seeing a therapist is beneficial at a particular time. We'll get to a more expansive questionnaire later in this chapter. For now, it may be helpful to keep in mind that if you can say yes to one or more of the following, therapy is definitely indicated: difficulty with core functioning, that is, feeding, watering, and/or sleeping; chronic irritability or just generally being "in a mood" to such a degree that trusted friends and family have started to gently (or not so gently) comment; little or no joy from activities, people, situations, and/or fandom attachments that once sparked a lot of joy; sudden emotions, meaning you are quick to cry, to get angry, to experience joy, etc.[ci]

How to Find a Therapist

Your best bet for finding a therapist who might be a good fit is to ask trusted people the name of their therapist and how they like them. Think Obi-Wan recommending his own "therapist," Yoda, to a young Luke Skywalker. We know that sometimes this conversation can feel a little awkward, but recall from the introduction the motto of the Starship Therapise: "verbalize to normalize." The more folks give voice to uncomfortable issues, the less uncomfortable they become. Another option is to look to online resources for therapists. The most widely used as of this writing is the website Psychology Today. But there are numerous sites that can be useful, particularly for marginalized folks. A couple of these include Inclusive Therapist, The Secular Therapy Project, and Melanin & Mental Health.

[ci] Basically, a lot of emotional quickness is happening.

Through these platforms, you can search for therapists in your area who fit criteria that you select, such as your potential therapist's gender, accepted insurance, treatment modality, and specialties. You can also find out whether this person is affirming or a member of marginalized groups such as people of color, LGBTQIA+ folks, the kink or BDSM community, folks with bigger bodies, etc. The one downside to using a website is that it can feel a little bit overwhelming at first. Utilizing the filters can help narrow it down a lot. Once you narrow down the search, read through your potential therapists' profiles and check out their respective websites. Make sure that you get a good sense of them and that you understand what kind of work they do. If you aren't sure, you can ask—seriously. Therapists need to be able to explain to you the kind of work they do and how they do it. If they can't, that's an indication that this probably isn't going to be your best therapist. When using a larger search engine like Psychology Today, you may notice that a high percentage of said photos are of white women. You might be wondering, *Why are so many therapists white women?* White folks have more access to advanced degrees because they have the social capital and momentum to afford graduate school as well as survive the often grueling prelicensure process, where pay is scant. Harkening back to chapter 2, recall that biological sex does not determine a person's gender expression. However, folks who are assigned female at birth and are then assigned the gender role of girl often gravitate toward helping fields. In America, as in many countries, folks raised as girls are taught to accommodate to and hold space for feelings, whereas those raised as boys are generally not. Additionally, with the exception of physicians, helping professionals tend to be compensated less than other specialists, in part because these jobs have historically been held by, and thus associated with, women.

Making First Contact

Once you've found one or more therapists who look like they might be a good fit, the next step is to reach out. On a website, there is typically an option to email or call potential therapists. In general, therapists use email to schedule sessions and phone, video, or in-office meetings to get into the why of therapy. But if you feel most comfortable briefly addressing the why in an email, that's fine too. Really, this stage is about setting up some type of direct exchange with a possible therapist so that you can start to get a sense of fit. And fit can be hard to describe. It's kind of like what happens when you just click with a new person. Is it because you both consider Frodo Baggins a personal hero? That's certainly part of it. But there's that other hard-to-quantify component that folks often describe as "vibing," "feeling comfortable," "being seen," or "not being judged." Think Luke when he first meets Obi-Wan, Captain Marvel when she meets Nick Fury,[242] or every Hogwarts student the first time they meet Albus Dumbledore. You need to directly engage with your prospective therapist to get a sense of this feeling.

When you reach out, ask if the person is taking on new clients. Yes, even if it looks like they are, they might not be. You may also want to ask if an initial consultation is free. Lots of folks will offer a fifteen-minute phone call just to get an idea of what's going on with you and whether they're skilled in that area. During the call, you can ask any questions you might have. Some specifics that you might want to know, if the information isn't easily found on the website, are the following:

- What are your rates?
- Do you take insurance?
- What style of therapy do you use, and what does that type of therapy look like?
- What are your favorite fandoms? If they don't know what you're talking about, that doesn't mean they aren't a good fit, but it does mean you might have to do some fandom education.

After you engage with your potential therapist and feel like it might be a good fit, you'll make your first appointment.

The First Session

Sometimes the first session is longer than future sessions so that you and your therapist can get to know each other a little better. Remember that getting to know your therapist will be different than getting to know a friend or colleague. The purpose of the relationship is for you to get your needs met, which means that most therapists won't tell you a ton about themselves. It's totally acceptable to ask questions, but be aware that your therapist might prefer not to answer if it feels too personal. Gandalf, Yoda, Professor X, and even Geralt of Rivia are selective about answering personal questions because their personal life isn't relevant to the quest. While this makes it tough to form reciprocal relationships with them, it is part of what makes them so sage-like: The sage archetype signifies a holder of wisdom and support.[243] They aren't there to be your new buddy. This may be the strangest thing about therapy. This person will know all of your innermost secrets, and you won't know much about them at all. But this is on purpose to help serve you best.

The first session(s) will include a lot of questions so that the therapist can get background information about you. It's always acceptable to not disclose things that feel too personal if you don't feel comfortable yet. And a good therapist will often lead with the reminder that just because they are asking you a question does not mean that you must answer it. In therapy, the client is the captain of the therapy ship, and the therapist is their support system. Unlike the Jedi Order, a therapist very much respects your consent and autonomy.

Hopefully you'll have a sense of whether your therapist is a good fit for you after this first session. But sometimes it can take a few sessions for you to be relaxed enough to pay much attention to what your therapist is doing. It's not uncommon to get caught up in your own head. You want a therapist who helps you feel safe enough to get uncomfortable. While Ciri and Geralt have a predominantly daughter-father relationship, Geralt also takes on the role of mentor. Young Ciri feels safe enough to try to learn to be a witcher—a grueling training process if there ever was one—because Geralt is a reassuring mentor. If after a few sessions you still don't feel like it's a good fit—in other words, you're feeling the opposite of safe with your therapist—then it might be time to seek out a new sage. Though it is normal to feel anxious about communicating this information, your therapist won't take it personally if you say you'd like to see someone else.

Ongoing Therapy

Once you find a therapist with whom you feel connected and want to continue working together, there are some more aspects to consider. It's important for your therapist to occasionally challenge you. If you notice that your therapist always agrees with and affirms you but never really challenges you, this might be an indication that you aren't moving through the stages of change. Mrs. Weasley, Ron's mom and supportive maternal figure to Harry, is great when it comes to reassurance and compassion. But she's not going to push Harry to change and grow as a wizard. Therapy needs to be uncomfortable sometimes because growing and changing are uncomfortable. It's a delicate balance of challenging and nurturing. Albus Dumbledore struggled with this balance too; he was constantly throwing his students into situations that were not developmentally appropriate. We're glad he wasn't Harry's therapist.

We invite you to ask your therapist for more challenges and to let them know when you feel like your needs aren't being met. There may be a reason that they're showing up in a certain way, such as the therapeutic model they use. The way you experience your therapist and therapy will have a lot to do with your therapist's skills, training, and style, i.e., the theories that inform their work. When you're a magician, there are many different types of magic and you get to decide your area of specialization.[cii] Are you a physical, psychic, illusions, healing, knowledge, or natural magician? It's often best to find a therapist whose specialization matches your needs. You wouldn't go to an herbalist if you need a psychic; that's just common sense. Ultimately, what feels the best to you and fits with your worldview is what is important.

The therapist's theoretical orientation can affect diagnostic labels, which refers to the name for the cluster of symptoms you experience.[244] Some theories stress the importance of diagnoses and some not at all. To our mind, labels are only as helpful as they feel to you, the client. Ultimately, you get to work together with your therapist to decide whether a diagnosis is meaningful for you.

[cii] Hat tip to *Burn Notice*. Magicians and spies have many things in common.

Types of Magic or Styles of Therapy

The following list is by no means exhaustive, but it gives you a good idea of the main therapeutic categories without getting too deep in the weeds. You'll also find some examples of therapist personality types mapped to each modality. And although not every CBT therapist is as much of a square as Faith's failed watcher Wesley Wyndam-Pryce, it will give you a general sense of what to expect from a therapist who practices each listed modality.

CBT (Cognitive Behavioral Therapy)[245]

If you change your behavior, you can change your thoughts. Or you can start with changing your thoughts and then change your behavior. Regardless, your mood should start to shift, and you'll start to feel better. Draco Malfoy could benefit from CBT; he has lots of problematic and frankly racist thoughts that cause him a ton of emotional distress, but he's not into the touchy-feely stuff. A CBT therapist could help Draco start to free himself from his negative cognitions through reality testing. The therapist might say something like, "I'm hearing how much you loathe Hermione Granger because of her intermagic heritage. What if you worked on a project together and you got the chance to reality-test your belief that all intermagic persons are inadequate?"

And what might a CBT provider look like? Think Wesley Wyndam-Pryce of *Buffy the Vampire Slayer* and *Angel* fame, but not the Wesley at the end of the *Angel* series: a roguish and wild man of questionable morals. No, we're talking the Wesley who appeared in *Buffy* with all of his straitlaced, rule-following glory. He was still delightful. He just had a very particular, rule-based worldview, which is somewhat common for a CBT therapist.

DBT (Dialectical Behavior Therapy)[246]

This style has four core tenets: mindfulness, distress tolerance, emotion regulation, and interpersonal effectiveness. DBT often involves both group and individual therapy. It was created by Marsha Linehan, a PhD who successfully copes with a serious and persistent mental illness. N'Jadaka, aka Erik Stevens, aka Killmonger, of *Black Panther*, struggles with violent mood swings, difficulty sustaining relationships, and an inaccurate perception of reality due to his history of significant trauma. If he'd had the ability to connect with others, a lot of what he experienced wouldn't have happened. A DBT therapist would help Erik to validate his concerns related to systemic racism while helping him practice emotion regulation and focusing on those things over which he does have control.

Pepper Potts of the MCU would make a great DBT therapist. She's a fan of order and structure while also understanding the importance of feelings.[247] Pepper would help you reality-test your way to a more regulated state using the tools of mindfulness and radical acceptance, while reminding you to validate your feelings. Your feelings are still real even when they don't fit the facts of the situation.

EMDR (Eye Movement Desensitization and Reprocessing)[248]

The crux of this style of therapy is rapid eye movement back and forth while recalling traumatic experiences. It's recommended for folks with both chronic and single-incident trauma, but its best outcomes are for folks with single-incident trauma. Gotham's Batman could use some EMDR to process the trauma of witnessing his parents' murder. Seeing a therapist would likely be a bit strange for Mr. Wayne, who is used to being very in control. The benefit of EMDR is that you get to decide how much (or how little) you disclose to your therapist. The important work is that you think of the traumatic event while doing the eye movements and following the protocol prompts from your therapist. It's sort of perfect for the untalkative Bruce (and some midwesterners). Once healed of his traumatic memories, Bruce could return to some of the activities that he once enjoyed and let go of trying to do anything and everything to numb out or make up for the trauma of watching his parents die.

Elliot Page in Christopher Nolan's *Inception*[249] is a great example of an EMDR therapist.[ciii] Think about it: they're helping clients to build a reality in which they can deal with their deepest darkest feelings, that is, reprocess their trauma. Not only that, but Elliot has a quality rapport with the folks

---

[ciii] And Leonardo DiCaprio's Cobb is a great example of an EMDR therapist suffering from empathy exhaustion and perhaps an undiagnosed substance-use disorder.

that they're working with, which is vital in EMDR work. Folks need to feel safe to reprocess trauma.

IFS (Internal Family Systems)[250]

In IFS, the therapist works from the assumption that none of us have a unitary consciousness, meaning that the human mind is made up of parts. This is actually quite intuitive. When you get invited to a party, a part of you wants to go and a part of you doesn't. IFS invites the client to talk to the parts from the Self, the director of the parts orchestra. Rogue, an X-Men with the power to absorb memories, feelings, and abilities from anyone she touches skin-to-skin, has many different parts of folks rolling around inside her brain. An IFS therapist would help Rogue to identify her Self among the sea of different people's parts and, from there, guide Rogue in learning how to talk with and lead these parts rather than having them lead her into dissociative identity disorder.

Professor X seems to be pretty into parts work—at least the traumatized emotional parts of his X-Men's minds. But, as we've mentioned, the professor has some boundary issues and also could work on his emotional intelligence. Perhaps that seems strange for a psychic, but think about all the times he encourages his X-Men pupils to just fight it out instead of being with their feelings. As he ages, Professor X gains in wisdom, so he'd be your ideal IFS therapist after doing his own IFS work. In fact, most IFS therapists are required to go through the IFS process before they can fully practice this modality. If you're looking for an IFS therapist, make sure to ask them if they've done their own IFS work. You want to make sure you're getting wise Professor X and not boy-genius Professor X.

Narrative Therapy[251]

It's the best style of therapy! We're kidding—sort of. We're clearly biased and like this style a lot. You read a little about it in chapter 1, so here's a brief refresher. Narrative therapy focuses on the importance of language and the story that people tell about their own lives. The most important belief in narrative therapy is that "the person is not the problem; the problem is the problem." Narrative therapists work with their clients to rewrite the stories of their life. Every case study you've seen has had elements of narrative therapy, so we won't offer another one. Obviously, we of the Starship Therapise are perfect examples of narrative therapists, but in case you need more examples we present to you Frodo Baggins. Frodo would make an empathic therapist who puts himself on the same level as his clients, never trying to tell them what to do, just working together to create a new story. He is able to separate the problem (the ring) from the person (everybody it possesses), and he could do the same with your problems.

Psychodynamic[252]

Psychodynamic therapy is the modern version of psychoanalytic therapy. It has elements of Freud and Jung on the whole conscious/unconscious thing but has pretty much let go of the sexy (Freud) god (Jung) stuff. Its main focus is to help increase your awareness around the unconscious or sublimated parts of your life experience so that you increase the control you have over your life. *The Legend of Zelda: Ocarina of Time*'s Ganon could really benefit from some psychodynamic work. He's clearly internalized a lot of negative feelings about being raised as a foundling in the desert while all the cool kids kicked it in Hyrule. But if you asked him why he's trying to take over Hyrule, he'd probably give you some line about absolute power and being a god[civ] yada-yada-yada. A psychodynamic therapist would validate these desires while encouraging Ganon to explore the roots of his lust for power.

Haku in *Spirited Away* would make an excellent psychodynamic therapist. He already has the training! He helps Chihiro, aka Sen, to make her way through the magical world (her unconscious) to find her way back to herself. He and Sen learn about themselves, with Chihiro helping Haku recover his lost name, allowing both of them to be freed from the unconscious forces that bind them. This is common in psychodynamic therapy, where transference and countertransference—your projection of unconscious parts onto your therapist and vice versa—allow the client to increase their awareness and can lead the therapist to increase their personal awareness too.

[civ] While we'd argue that archetypes could be very helpful in working with Ganon (god complex much?), a psychodynamic therapist probably wouldn't go there.

Family Systems Therapy[253] (aka Marriage and Family Therapy)

Since we've already learned a lot about this modality in chapters 7 and 8, we're not going to spend too much extra time here. Family systems therapy looks at the impact that your different families—family of origin and families of choice—have on your life. Psychodynamic therapy overlaps with family therapy in that both schools believe that our early familial experiences become internalized and show up for us in life, often in ways we aren't conscious of at first. Similar to narrative therapy, all of the case studies in this book incorporate aspects of family systems, with chapter 8's *Rocinante* crew being the canonical example. You know who else could really benefit from this therapeutic approach? Wolverine, aka Logan. While he likes to think of himself as a lone wolf(erine), he is profoundly impacted by his traumatic family of origin story and his problematic family of sort-of choice, the Weapon X program. Logan's family systems therapist would do well to start slow and focus on gaining his trust by validating his loner skills and highlighting his successful turn as an X-Men team member before suggesting a family therapy session with adopted daughters Jubilee, Kitty Pryde, Laura Kinney, problematic pseudobrother Victor Creed, and father figure Professor X.

But who would lead this therapy? None other than Counselor Troi. Think about it: not only is Deanna Troi an empath, but she's also done a lot of her own personal work to better understand her family.[cv] She knows how to support and validate all kinds of different familial systems while challenging different family members when needed. Just think about all those gentle heart-to-hearts with Captain Picard. He didn't want to go to therapy. But Counselor Troi used some good old-fashioned Rogerian[cvi] unconditional positive regard coupled with Sal Minuchin's structural family therapy approaches to meet Picard where he was and then gently push him into change.

—

[cv] An entire year could be devoted to mom Lwaxana Troi alone.

[cvi] Carl Rogers believed that healing comes from unconditional positive regard. He was like the Jim Henson of therapy.

Now, let's circle back to your musings from the start of the chapter. Take out your ponderings and peruse them. Notice how you feel toward these thoughts now, without assigning any judgment. Do you feel the same or differently than you did a little while ago? All answers are welcome. If your views have started to shift, then you've practiced some Therapeutic Fanfiction without even really trying, friends. That's the power of this model.

Question Yourself

As promised, here is a self-care questionnaire that can help you to determine if now is the right time to seek out your Jedi Master, aka your own therapist. Please note that this scale is not a clinical diagnostic instrument and is provided for educational purposes only.[cvii] So take out your quills or magic pens and fill this out.

SELF-CARE QUESTIONNAIRE[cviii]

Instructions: Circle the answer that is most true for you in the past month (unless otherwise noted). Tally your score when complete.

1. I have at least one full day off work each week.
   (0) Never / (1) Seldom / (2) Sometimes / (3) Often / (4) Always
2. I take some time for myself daily to be quiet, think, meditate, and/or write.
   (0) Never / (1) Seldom / (2) Sometimes / (3) Often / (4) Always
3. I work fewer than ten hours per day.
   (0) Never / (1) Seldom / (2) Sometimes / (3) Often / (4) Always

---

[cvii] Again, we are not your therapists, unless of course we are your therapists.

[cviii] Adapted from the "Self-Care and Lifestyle Balance Inventory," Headington Institute (2020).

4. I mindfully move my body doing something I enjoy (running, yoga, Zumba, hiking, tap dancing, etc.) at least two times per week.
(0) Never / (1) Seldom / (2) Sometimes / (3) Often / (4) Always

5. I give myself permission to play (video or tabletop gaming, Netflix binges, coloring) at least two times per week.
(0) Never / (1) Seldom / (2) Sometimes / (3) Often / (4) Always

6. I practice mindfulness, meditation, or deep breathing daily.
(0) Never / (1) Seldom / (2) Sometimes / (3) Often / (4) Always

7. I share how I am feeling with at least one friend or my partner daily.
(0) Never / (1) Seldom / (2) Sometimes / (3) Often / (4) Always

8. I sleep well and feel rested in the morning.
(0) Never / (1) Seldom / (2) Sometimes / (3) Often / (4) Always

9. I eat foods that I enjoy and that give me energy.
(0) Never / (1) Seldom / (2) Sometimes / (3) Often / (4) Always

10. I drink at least eight eight-ounce (8 oz) glasses of water a day.
(0) Never / (1) Seldom / (2) Sometimes / (3) Often / (4) Always

11. I have more positive emotional experiences than negative.
(0) Never / (1) Seldom / (2) Sometimes / (3) Often / (4) Always

12. I have separate time for work and play and feel solid about that separation.
(0) Never / (1) Seldom / (2) Sometimes / (3) Often / (4) Always

13. I recognize when I'm becoming tired, rundown, and vulnerable to illness.
(0) Never / (1) Seldom / (2) Sometimes / (3) Often / (4) Always

14. I surround myself with people who care about me, whom I trust, and whom I can talk to if I choose.
(0) Never / (1) Seldom / (2) Sometimes / (3) Often / (4) Always

15. I engage in creative or expressive activities (such as writing or painting) at least one time per week.
(0) Never / (1) Seldom / (2) Sometimes / (3) Often / (4) Always

16. I set and maintain healthy boundaries for myself, saying "no" when I need to.
(0) Never / (1) Seldom / (2) Sometimes / (3) Often / (4) Always

17. When I am working, I give myself permission to take breaks.
(0) Never / (1) Seldom / (2) Sometimes / (3) Often / (4) Always

18. I spend time with trusted others who are part of a community of meaning and purpose (activist organizations, clubs, volunteers, teams, virtual communities) at least once per week.
(0) Never / (1) Seldom / (2) Sometimes / (3) Often / (4) Always

19. I am able to communicate what I mean effectively with others.
(0) Never / (1) Seldom / (2) Sometimes / (3) Often / (4) Always

20. I feel good about how I spend my time or energy relative to what is really important to me in life.
(0) Never / (1) Seldom / (2) Sometimes / (3) Often / (4) Always

21. I show myself the same compassion that I show others.
(0) Never / (1) Seldom / (2) Sometimes / (3) Often / (4) Always

22. I set realistic goals for myself and give myself positive messages about my ability to accomplish them—even when I encounter difficulties.
(0) Never / (1) Seldom / (2) Sometimes / (3) Often / (4) Always

23. I take days off from work when I need to due to illness, family obligations, empathy exhaustion, etc.
(0) Never / (1) Seldom / (2) Sometimes / (3) Often / (4) Always

24. I am able to let go of mistakes I have made.
(0) Never / (1) Seldom / (2) Sometimes / (3) Often / (4) Always

25. I am able to manage conflict constructively, that is, without it boiling over into fights with others and without stuffing my feelings just to "get along."
(0) Never / (1) Seldom / (2) Sometimes / (3) Often / (4) Always

26. I am able to let go of grudges.
(0) Never / (1) Seldom / (2) Sometimes / (3) Often / (4) Always

27. I feel comfortable with my relationship to drugs and alcohol.
(0) Never / (1) Seldom / (2) Sometimes / (3) Often / (4) Always

Total Score: ______

INTERPRETATION GUIDELINES

0–27:
A score in this range suggests a danger of burnout and a general lack of self-care. As Saru on *Star Trek Discovery* once famously said to his friend and colleague Tilly, "You're important too." The time to find your therapist is now!

28–54:
A score in this range suggests that your self-care skills and lifestyle-balance strategies could use improvement. Although reaching out to a therapist isn't mission critical, it definitely needs to be moved to the top five on your to-do list.

55–81:
A score in this range suggests that you have spent some time working on yourself and that you have tools to cope with mild-to-moderate life stressors. But it seems like when stress is high that you could benefit from some additional support.

82 AND ABOVE:
A score in this range suggests that you have established self-care skills and lifestyle-balance strategies and maintain them effectively. You may already have a therapist or supportive mentor in your life! If you have neither but feel like you would like one, now might be the time to find your watcher. We can almost always benefit from a Giles.

11

A Swiftly Tilting Planet: Saving Earth

Frodo: I wish the ring had never come to me.
I wish none of this had ever happened.

Gandalf: So do all who live to see such times,
but that is not for them to decide. All we have to decide
is what to do with the time that is given to us.

—*THE LORD OF THE RINGS: THE FELLOWSHIP OF THE RING*[254]

We started writing this book before the pandemic of 2020 hit North America. Although we had always planned a chapter to focus on the world in which we live, the place that makes all life possible, our planet Earth, we could not have foreseen some of the events that have made life on Earth increasingly precarious. We spent time in chapter 2 exploring the continued impact of systemic oppression and injustice, and here we will focus on the sociopolitical and economic forces destroying the planet. You can't rewrite your life if you have nowhere to live it.

It's important to know that some—or all—of the topics discussed herein might cause discomfort. They might bring up feelings of pain, sadness, anger, loss, and/or disappointment. You might therefore ask yourself,

Couldn't I just skip ahead to chapter 12? Well, you could. But we invite you to stay. Part of Therapeutic Fanfiction involves sitting with hard truths because sitting with this discomfort helps us make important and sometimes life-altering changes. Remember the Mirror of Erised from *Harry Potter and the Philosopher's Stone*? For those who need a recap, Harry, an orphan who has been the victim of intrafamily violence and abuse throughout his childhood, gets invited to study at a magic boarding school, Hogwarts School of Witchcraft and Wizardry. During his first term, Harry stumbles upon said mirror that will show the gazer that which they most desire. So, when Harry looks in the mirror, he sees himself surrounded by his long-dead parents and the extended family that might have been. When Harry looks in the mirror and sits with his feelings of grief and loss, he is able to realize how much he wants a family. He uses this knowledge to help him build a family of choice, first with Hagrid, then Ron, and, at last, Hermione. In fact, the entire series charts, among other things, Harry's journey to co-create that which he saw in the mirror: a family. Without looking at this hard truth straight in the face, Harry might have held onto his grief without the insight into what he needed to make it better.

In the case of our IRL events, it can be easy to slide into a pit of despair, ruing what has happened to our beloved rock. But as we look our reality in the face, we are able to grapple both with climate collapse, the rise of communicable diseases like COVID-19, and what control we have to make changes and fanfic our world.

Let's pause for a moment and sit with the feelings that are coming up right now. You have skills to draw on to help you sit with this discomfort. And once you're feeling a bit calmer, do some thinking or journaling around your feelings on the state of the Earth, the pandemic, and whatever else the beginning of this chapter evoked for you. Remember that you are not sitting with these truths alone; we are right here with you.

Death, Part 1: Sitting with Hard Truths

We thought we would get arguably the most challenging uncomfortable truth done right away. No time like the present! Because, literally, it's all we have. Time is a construct. The hard truth is in order to stay alive, something else has to die. And we don't mean a tit-for-tat type situation. We're talking literally a cow has to die to make your cheeseburger. Or a carrot has to die to make your carrot cake. We are not making value judgments on anyone's eating choices. This is not a book about how it's "better" or more "moral" to be a vegan vs. a vegetarian vs. an omnivore. This is a book about mindful awareness.

Since the dawn of human thought, or since as far back as we have cave paintings, humans have been struggling with this central tension between life and death. Joseph Campbell wrote a very long book about it. Well, he wrote several. But one of the longest, *Primitive Mythology,* volume 1 of *The Masks of God,* explored early humanity's struggle to reconcile death with life. Vampires are a great example of this concept. Whether it's *True Blood, Twilight, Fledgling, Interview with the Vampire,* or *What We Do in the Shadows,* our pale friends are constantly worried about what they eat and how they get it. Is it OK to eat people? Some vamps like Lestat à la *Interview with the Vampire* and the *What We Do in the Shadows* crew say yea! Some, like *Twilight*'s tortured Edward, say nay. No doubt after noting the references to early humanity's cannibalism,[cix] Campbell would remind us that vampire stories are just one of many examples of humanity grappling with the discomfort we feel about eating other creatures and plants to stay alive. This discomfort has bothered humanity all the way up to present day, and we've used the powers of Therapeutic Fanfiction to write all sorts of stories to distance ourselves from this reality and assuage any potential guilt.

Modern humans usually center these stories around the idea that some life is just more lively than other life. In other words, human life is more valuable or worthy or important than other types of life, such as your dog or your cat or Bessie the cow or that oak tree your grandfather used to swing on. Does this sound familiar? If you're a fan of *Westworld,* then it sure does.

The reason we invite you to sit with the reality that life must consume other life to live is that it opens up our awareness to another insight: all life is valuable. Part of the reason we have put life into a hierarchical pyramid is to justify (i.e., help ourselves feel better about) consuming other life. But

---

[cix] Yep, it's documented. History—it's great.

we can both value all life and recognize that we need to consume some of it sometimes to maintain our own life. Now more than ever, it is crucial that human beings learn to sit with these unpleasant truths because our old story about some life being more valuable than other life has enabled humanity to make decisions that are killing the planet.

Let's pause. First, you're doing a great job of sitting with hard truths. We're proud of you. Second, now might be a solid time to express or write down some of the feelings that have come up for you thus far. Even though that was only one section, it was a lot. We invite you to engage and identify your feelings rather than judge them. Reflect back to what you wrote at the start of the chapter: are new thoughts already coming to you? If so, that makes sense. You are starting the Therapeutic Fanfiction process, which requires a lot of revision. If you don't have anything new coming up, that's just fine too. Let us continue forth, hero.

Death Part 2: Guilt and Shame

Now that you've jotted down more thoughts, let's have a look at what you've written. Without judgment, notice how you speak about yourself. It's possible that you are experiencing some shame around your impact on the Earth and the Earth's flora and fauna. All feelings are welcome. Did you know that there's a small but important difference between guilt and shame? Let's recall the fanfic case study from chapter 6: Dean Winchester. Dean expresses feelings that he doesn't deserve care and attention. Some of his beliefs formed because for a time Dean was a torturer in literal Hell. He believes that he is a bad person because of this role. When he expresses this to his brother Sam, the very tall little brother doesn't believe Dean is a bad person; he believes Dean is a good person who did a bad thing. Recall from chapter 4 that every feeling has a core message and a corresponding call to action. Guilt's core message lets you know that you have shirked your responsibility, and the call to action is to make amends.[255] Shame's core message is that you've done something so heinous and unforgivable as to be no longer fit for society. The call to action is to thus hide whatever you've done to trigger this shame so as not to be excommunicated from your social group. Feeling like a bad person is shame; feeling like a good (or neutral) person who did a bad thing is guilt. Some guilt is healthy; shame, however, doesn't really help you to move forward. As long as you live in a state of shame, you will not be able to face yourself or your decisions. Shame makes change impossible.

Apologies for the Apocalypse

Your thoughts and feelings around climate change, where the COVID-19 pandemic came from, and why certain policy leaders are in charge are based on your Westworld Constructs. Remember that the Westworld Construct is a malleable tool, so consider which of your beliefs are serving you and greater society and which are not.

As a story-loving species, we have been exploring what it would mean to face the end of modern life as we know it for generations. The post-apocalyptic genre is compelling because it invites us to be fanfic writers and to mentally prepare for all that may come. In most of our fandom favorites, there's a great divide before finally coming together. Think of the districts in *The Hunger Games*[256] or the factions in the *Divergent* series[257] or the caste system in N. K. Jemisin's *The Broken Earth* series. All these books show a future in which humans are divided and must come together for survival. Perhaps none track this journey more poignantly than *The Broken Earth* trilogy. Divided by betrayal and the Earth itself, the mother and daughter Essun and Nassun must decide how and if to save the world.[258]

Zombies are another popular modern metaphor for the demise of our way of life post–Industrial Revolution. Whether you're a *Walking Dead* head, *Parable of the Sower*[259] lit nerd,[cx] *Dawn of the Dead* aficionado, or a *Last of Us* gamer, zombies resonate with you perhaps because, among other things, they are an excellent metaphor for viral plague. And what do the people in those stories do? They fight back in whatever way they can,

---

[cx] Although the series was initially conceived as a triptych, Octavia E. Butler never completed it, in part due to the systemic racism and sexism she regularly experienced as an African American woman writing science fiction in the 1980s and 1990s.

before ultimately succumbing to the futility of trying to defeat a zombie foe. We offer that this is due in large part to what the zombie symbolizes: You can no more fight a virus using strength and will power than you can defeat a mob of zombies with gumption and a baseball bat with nails. Zombies usually aren't defeated; you just have to get rid of enough of them so there aren't as many to fight and keep folks from getting turned. Does that sound like a killer metaphor for social distancing and herd immunity?

Vampires, zombies, and postapocalyptic stories are all ways that we've been trying to cope with and better understand our dying planet and hostile viruses. We can use these stories and the awareness brought to us by the Westworld Construct to begin to chart a course to fight for the future. That brings us to another apocalyptic fandom story: *Outer Wilds*.

The Eye of the Universe

If you haven't played this game, we can't recommend it highly enough. In *Outer Wilds*, your avatar is a kind, gender-nonbinary alien of the Hearthian people. When the game opens, you're about to go on your first ever space mission.[260] You say goodbye to your Hearthian pals, get a gentle info drop about the Nomai—an ancient alien race that traveled the galaxy in search of something called "the eye of the universe" before they all inexplicably died out ages ago—and you set off . . . only to die within twenty-two minutes of game play. When your avatar wakes up, you find yourself back on your home planet about to start your first ever space mission. And the game just continues on these twenty-two-minute cycles as you attempt to search your small home solar system for answers to this life-death loop that you're stuck in.

Outer Wilds provides a template for many things, not the least of which is how to grapple with death mindfully. All emotions have a call to action, and the bigger or more intense the feeling, the louder the internal call to act. *Outer Wilds* harnesses this intense call to action through the death loop; nothing like a twenty-two-minutes-to-live time crunch to really get you motivated to look for answers. The game taps into our desire to live and to see our community survive.

Early thinkers like John Locke and Thomas Hobbes pushed the idea that human beings are driven by just one desire: to live and thrive at all costs. And while we salute Locke and Hobbes for trying, we and many others—Carl Jung, Joseph Campbell, Melanie Klein, Virginia Satir, and Kimberlé Williams Crenshaw—offer that they missed a few things: play, for one; the desire for community, for another; and auxiliary drives like art, love, and spirituality. One of the primal tensions for humanity has been the tension between the individual and the community. What happens when what you want or need conflicts with what your community wants or needs? Do we always agree with Spock that the needs of the many outweigh the needs of the few?

Outer Wilds resolves this conflict by postulating two alien races for whom individuality and connection harmonize. The Nomais are a race of explorers; each individual is driven by equal parts curiosity and compassion. The Hearthians are an alien race that more closely resembles what we think of in modern Earthen times as a large extended family. In this society, each member performs the role that best matches their skill set. Think of it like an orchestra or a band. Each Hearthian finds their own personal instrument to play together with their other orchestra or band members, and it is together that they are able to create wonderful music. Locke[261] and Hobbes[262] would argue that a sentient being's ultimate self-expression is to kill all the other band members and play a riotous solo on the charred remains. And while we agree that such a solo would be good—horrific but certainly good—there's just no way it rivals the result of everyone playing together at peak self-expression.

Part of what we want to encourage you to do with this book, reader, is to question the status quo. And that includes the status quos of religion; social systems policing bodies, races, and ethnicity; governments; and political structures. We certainly don't claim to have all the answers. But this idea that human beings are fundamentally self-serving and in an unending cycle of competition to be king of death mountain? We couldn't reject that more if we tried. Life challenges you to explore many different ways to perceive your world and grow within it. While we don't ask that you join us in rejecting the king of death-mountain construct, we do ask that you engage with it and get curious about other options.

Now back to feelings. All roads lead back to these troublesome sensations that are the building blocks of our connection with one another, other creatures, and our planet. Play is how we shift from emotions and intelligence to perception and planning. Play is fundamental both to how we learn and process what we perceive in our internal and external realities. Playing a game like *Outer Wilds*[cxi] can help you learn how to sit with hard truths and big feelings like death and sadness. It can also help you learn how to meditate; we'll talk about this more in our fanfic case study. Play can help you figure out what to do when those feelings call you to action. Just like in *Outer Wilds*, our planet is dying. Life as we know it is ending. And there are things we can do about it!

General Grievous

Grief, the final frontier, is arguably the most challenging of all emotional processes. It's why so many humans avoid it.[263] Grief is a universal human experience. Even if someone close to you has not been very ill or not passed away, you've felt grief over other losses in your life. It can be harder to pinpoint these, because unlike the death of a loved one, it's harder to point to one reason for your sadness.[264] Therapists call this kind of grief ambiguous loss. Let's pause for a moment and check in with ourselves.

Reflect in your mind palace or on paper about the losses you've experienced, whether they be the physical loss of a loved one or some other loss, such as a relationship, a career, or a dream from your youth. Once you've reflected, consider how you're feeling toward these losses now. If you think to yourself, *I wish I wasn't upset about that,* consider what you would say to a friend struggling with the same thing. We suspect that you would offer that other human compassion. Can you do the same for yourself?

Let's recall the most visceral of all *Buffy the Vampire Slayer* episodes: "The Body."[265] In the episode, Buffy Summers's mother, Joyce, dies, and

---

[cxi] For those of you who are really into video game research, *Outer Wilds* has pitch perfect ludonarrative resonance. *Ludonarrative* refers to the interaction between the story of a video game and the gaming mechanics, i.e., the way your avatar progresses through the game.

viewers see each character's own journey through grief. This episode does a lovely job of exploring how people experience grief differently. According to Elisabeth Kübler-Ross, there are five stages of grief: denial, anger, bargaining, depression, and acceptance.[266] Growing evidence suggests a sixth stage centered around meaning-making, clearly influenced by the work of Viktor Frankl, put forth by Kübler-Ross's longtime collaborator David Kessler.[267] These stages do not happen in any kind of linear fashion, nor do they end, exactly. When you grieve, you move through each of these stages in various orders, each time resting in acceptance a little bit longer. If you permit yourself to grieve, you will eventually make your way to acceptance and hang out there most of the time. Inevitably, an event will occur in daily life that brings you back to loss, and then you will recycle through these stages. This process of grieving acutely, resting in acceptance, and returning to grief continues indefinitely.

When different people grieve, they can be in different stages at the same time. This helps explain the difficulties that often ensue between family members during the loss of a loved one. For example, it can feel alienating, frustrating, and just generally upsetting when you are in the stage of depression while a fellow family member is in the bargaining stage, trying to convince you that your terminally ill loved one is "going to make it somehow." We can use the stages of grief model to help us understand the many disparate reactions to the climate crisis. Folks struggling to accept the reality of the planet's demise are in the denial stage. Mindful awareness can help you to step back and give yourself and your fellow humans space to be with their respective feelings and stage of grief.

We become frustrated in life when reality doesn't match our expectations, so if we expect that we will experience one feeling per week for five weeks and then we're all better, that isn't going to end well emotionally. But if we know that it will take time and won't be linear, and will be difficult, then we can have more compassion for ourselves.[cxii]

[cxii] Incidentally, if you want to watch a character rapidly move through the stages of grief in one therapy session, *The OC* has a great episode: "The Metamorphosis," where Summer Roberts does just that.

Caring for a Changing World

The planet is dying.[268] The way that human beings have been living and working post–Industrial Revolution has been decimating the earth's ecosystems and atmosphere. We are not looking to shame folks who've come before us and made those choices. They were doing the best they knew how to do at the time. What we are doing is inviting those who know better to do better. We know more now. And that knowledge—and the related feelings—calls us to action. We have until 2030 to make broad, sweeping systemic changes to help stave off total climate demise. So, as great as it is to cut down on your personal consumption and do things like give up plastic straws, we need far-reaching communal action to change our collective fates.

Let's pause. Just be with the feelings coming up for you. Without judgment, notice what stage of grief is the most present right now. Simply let it be there. Perhaps reflect or journal, or maybe even draw or make crafts, and then come back to this chapter in a little bit.

Thus far, we've spent some time detailing the shitty wrapping of this gift. We promise there's a gift here. And the gift is . . . you. Perhaps you're thinking, *But you just said we can't do this individually!* Yes, and change almost always starts with a spark. As we've discussed throughout this book, human beings are designed to be sensitive creatures. Our human bodies and minds help us to tune into the world around us and to then communicate what we're perceiving to others. Fandom, play, and stories have power because they make us feel, and feelings are the building blocks of change. If you've felt impacted by anything you've read in here, you are going to go out into the world and effect change. Put another way, every rock you toss in water has ripples. And hundreds of thousands of ripples can make a wave. And what humanity needs is a tsunami if we are going to shift course and save ourselves and our planet.

What does this change look like in practice? It can look like all kinds of things. You're already changing and embodying this change by reading this book and talking about it with yourself and others. You are enacting microactivism, which becomes macro as it moves ever outward. *Captain Planet and the Planeteers*, the 1990s American cartoon, encouraged an entire generation of American kids to recycle.[269] Perhaps some of you recall that recycling initiatives were partially funded and propagated by large businesses to mitigate the public anxiety about excess waste and to encourage continued consumption because, "Hey, everything can just be recycled!" Well, those are hard facts too.[270]

But there's hope here. In the 1970s, people were collectively starting to feel anxious about the planet because we are hardwired to respond to our external environment, aka planet Earth. We numb out or reach for denial because, as human beings, we tend to care too much and don't always know how to be with those feelings. The genius of a show like *Captain Planet* is that it helped young humans feel inspired and empowered to help their planet and their community. It gave a story and a voice to an issue that made sense to people, instead of previous attempts that tried to evoke feelings of shame to encourage behavior change.[cxiii] We aren't motivated by shame, as we've seen, because shame overwhelms our brains and bodies with messages saying that we are so flawed as to be beyond repair. In response, humans attempt to run from that which is causing the feeling of shame rather than fight to change it, because shame says that all efforts are futile. But you can't outrun your feelings; they're always trailing right behind you. *Captain Planet* taught children that they have a responsibility to the planet and attempted to give children concrete tools to care for the Earth. Therapeutic Fanfiction invites you to put this "problem" on your fellowship vision board and pair it with an inspirational fandom character. Perhaps yours is Captain Planet, but maybe it's Summer Roberts from *The OC* when she gets real political[271] or some other character. If you can write a narrative in your life where you choose to make an impact and share your story, then you can be the spark of change that can grow into a collective movement.

The following is a list of ways to consider for challenging existing Westworld Constructs:

- Bring awareness to the ways that you make clothing purchases. Are we saying to never shop fast fashion again? Not necessarily, but we are inviting you to think about the impact that your shopping habits

---

[cxiii] Please see "The Crying Indian" commercials of the 1970s.

have both on yourself and the human collective. Living in a late-stage capitalist society means facing these kinds of questions and challenges regularly. We also invite you to consider other products you buy, where they come from, how they're made and tested, and how they get to you.

- Bring awareness to kinds and types of food; who harvests, ships, and prepares food; as well as the environmental imprint of meat vs. plant-based foods. This has nothing to do with body sizes. It's about critically engaging with that age-old tension between life and death. As an example, the more we are able to sit with our love for bacon and our respect for the sentience of pigs, the more we will be able to make decisions that acknowledge both feelings.
- Verbalize to normalize. We've used this phrase before; in this context, we deploy it as a fanfiction call to action! Share with others your thoughts and feelings related to ethical consumption. Share with others your struggles with politics, race, and gender roles. It's not about sharing answers but rather inviting friends into the process of increased awareness and critical inquiry.
- Ask for help and support. Sitting with the realities of a shifting planet is challenging. Charles Wallace, one of the three protagonists in Madeleine L'Engle's original trilogy, consisting of *A Wrinkle in Time*, *A Wind in the Door*, and *A Swiftly Tilting Planet*, needed a lot of help from a variety of folks—family, friends, aliens—to save the planet. Once he got over his boy-genius self, he was able to use his words to *ask* for this help.[272] Turning to loved ones whom you can trust to process the realities of climate collapse or global consumer greed can help to stave off feelings of shame and helplessness, while reminding you that you aren't alone in this.
- Radical acceptance toward action. Once you start sitting with our global challenges, global inequalities, and global atrocities, you can start to lose hope. You might also struggle with nihilism, or the idea that nothing matters. Radical acceptance can help. Radical acceptance invites you to accept forces that are actually beyond your control, thus helping you to clearly see where you do have control.

- Mobilize your fellowship. Find a like-minded group of individuals and mobilize. These are systemic problems, and for change to happen we must work together to demand swift and effective action. As Galadriel said, "Even the smallest person can change the course of the future,"[273] yet even Frodo needed his fellowship. We can do great things if we do them together. So find your IRL fellowship, coordinate with other fellowships, and start demanding change from the systems perpetuating systemic oppression and global annihilation. Multinational corporations are not going to change themselves.

You're starting to pull together all the skills you need to rewrite your life, and the pale blue dot where you live is a vital part of this process. We invite you to consider how you make meaning from all of this information, even when you know that you can't control all aspects of your world. Can you find meaning in those things you can control? It can help to embrace the choices you do have, as Frankl taught: a person can survive any *how* for a *why*. The knowledge of finality is what helps us make meaning, perhaps because grappling with loss is so painful. After all, magic comes from pain. Think of the final episodes of *The Good Place*.[274] The six friends finally make it to the real good place but find it unfulfilling. Everything Eleanor, Chidi, Tahani, Jason, Michael, and Janet could ever want is available to them forever. Their afterlives feel devoid of meaning because there is no end to joy and there is no goal to work toward. Human beings and demons alike thrive when they have goals and the possibility for transcendence. *The Good Place* pals find meaning in utopia when they realize that they can create a system that helps all beings—human, angelic, and demonic—to continue growing and changing on an everlasting journey to become their highest selves.

The Earth has never seen a collective system that helps all human beings grow, change, and learn to become their highest selves. But just because we haven't gotten there doesn't mean we can't! If we can all work together, this place can be the good place.

Where do we go from here? As we conclude this chapter, we invite you to return to the example of *Outer Wilds*, a game that explores the central tension between individual growth and communal change. No matter how hard your avatar works, they are unable to prevent the death of the universe in which they and their community lives. Yet through your avatar's journey that they are able to triumph where the more technologically advanced Nomai failed: your avatar enters the eye of the universe, and the universe itself is reborn. The hero's journey must conclude with a return to community, where the hero can present the gift they achieved on their adventure, thereby helping all beings. We may not always know how or when our story will end. But with the power of choice and the gifts from our adventures, we can ensure that other stories continue and begin long after ours has ended.

Self, the Final Frontier

As we grapple with the catastrophes of the twenty-first century, it may be helpful to reflect on the thinkers of the twentieth century who faced the horrors of WWII and the atrocities of modern colonialism.[275] They asked the question: why, with all of the advances of technology, was humanity sinking ever deeper into oppression, racism, and the ruin of the natural world due to industrialization? Where was utopia? Though we certainly don't claim to know the formula for economic utopia, we offer that one of the answers to these questions centers around the relationship between individual and communal emotional awareness. As a species, we have prioritized technological growth over emotional growth, and it shows. The challenge for those of us in the twenty-first century is the journey of the self.

Remember that quote from *Star Trek: The Next Generation*'s Q way back at the start of the book? Here's a refresher: "That is the exploration that awaits you: not mapping stars and studying nebula but charting the unknown possibilities of existence."[276] We keep looking *out there*, but what we really need to do is to look *in here*, inside ourselves. If each of us can work on exploring our personal selves, understanding our feelings, and learning new ways to engage collectively, then perhaps we will be able to discover, if not utopia, at least a kinder and more compassionate way to exist together.

FANFIC CASE STUDY:
Outer Wilds, Living a Full Life in Twenty-Two Minutes or Less

After a brief but rousing sojourn in the realm of teletherapy, we decide to return to in-person therapy sessions. At least, this was the plan. We run into some difficulties with our new intake, Gabbro of the Hearthian people, who is marooned on a distant planet in a far-flung galaxy. To make things even more complicated, Gabbro is caught in a time loop in which they and their galaxy die at the end of twenty-two minutes, only to have everything restored when the time loop starts up again. Needless to say, we are intrigued. After talking with Starfleet about the option of taking a shuttle craft to the eye of the universe and having this option strongly vetoed by the admiralty (something about it being "possibly against the prime directive"[cxiv] and "endangering the timeline" not to mention risking "two of Starfleet's best and brightest"), a work-around is devised: we will beam virtual projections of ourselves down to the planet, Giant's Deep, to meet our new client, Gabbro.

Today, the morning of our first session with Gabbro, dawns bright and hopeful. After a breakfast of champions—waffles with whipped cream and strawberries for Kirk and a vegetarian egg-white omelet for Spock—we cue up the transporter and virtually beam ourselves down to the surface of Giant's Deep. After a brief hike and dodging the tempestuous waves of the planet (Gabbro warned us it was 50 percent water, and they did not exaggerate), we find our newest client lying in a hammock, staring up at the sky with an instrument at their right side.

"Hello," we wave, approaching the hammock. "You must be Gabbro."

"Oh yes, the therapists! You made it and with seventeen minutes to spare. That'll at least give us some time to get acquainted before . . ." Gabbro trails off, still staring up at the gray sky. We note that they haven't

[cxiv] The Starfleet rule forbids interference in other species' growth and development.

made eye contact even once since our arrival. "Have you accounted for the time loop?"

We answer, "Yes, we'll be able to meet you back here each time your memories are sent back in time."

Gabbro nods. "To another version of me. Yes, I see. It's strange, isn't it? Dying every time. And when I come to, I think I'm still me. But I'm past me with future me's memories—a whole series of future me's."

"Of course, that would be so difficult. How do you cope with it all?" we ask.

"At first, I tried playing my Hearthian flute. That helped, actually. It's the thing I did when I was just a hatchling, to comfort myself."

"That makes a lot of sense and was so intuitive. Great awareness, Gabbro!"

"Oh, thank you. It's so nice to talk to someone. It feels like it's been . . . well, longer than twenty-two minutes." For the first time, Gabbro glances at us. We can't quite make out their eyes through the glint off their helmet, but the shift of their head makes even a moment's worth of eye contact more likely than not. "I just don't know if I can keep doing this—dying and not dying. It's wrecking even the twenty-two minutes I've got because all I can think about is how close the end is. And the panic . . . it's unbearable."

"Of course it is, Gabbro. What you're experiencing is something called anticipatory distress. You are so worried about the events to come that you can't focus on what is happening right now in front of you, not to mention that you have all of those memories tapping into your grief. You have so much going on that your brain is being pulled in two directions, memories of the past and fears of the future. There's no space for the present."

"Yes, that's exactly it!" exclaims Gabbro, sitting up in the hammock. "And I want to be able to be in the present. It's all I have."

"That's right. All any of us have is now. Let's talk a little bit about how to stay in the now, shall we?"

"Yeah. Yeah, all right. I think that sounds really good."

"This might sound a little strange and definitely feel a little strange at first, but just roll with us. Bring your awareness to your breath. There's no need to control your breathing, just notice what the air feels like as the air comes in . . . and goes out . . ."

Gabbro folds their legs up underneath them and takes a deep breath in and then, after a few moments, exhales deeply. They take a few more breaths and say, "All right, yeah. I think that is helping. I can feel my heart slow and the pressure in my chest is definitely going down. Hmm. I suppose I could just do that for twenty-two minutes. But the thing is, I also want to be able to do other things. Like radio to Hornfels or play my flute. Maybe even have a snack."

"Of course, that makes sense. This is just an exercise to help you feel more present. What you do with that presence is up to you. As you go about your twenty-two minutes, if you notice that your mind is starting to run away with memories from the past or worries for the future, you can again focus on your breath until the panic starts to dissipate. This is called mindfulness. When you engage in this sort of mindfulness while you sit and focus on your breath, you are engaging in meditation."

"I like it. Hmm."

"Is something coming up?"

"Well, I was just thinking that I wish there was something I could do. I already tried radioing to Hornfels about the whole time-loop thing, but, so far, they haven't taken me seriously. When I'm not panicking, I hate thinking about all my friends so close to death and not even knowing. I want to tell them."

"How would that help?"

"I think maybe if I told them we could find some way to work together to save our planet, to save the whole solar system. I can't do it all by myself. But I know we could do it together." Then Gabbro becomes very still. For a few moments, we wonder if they are even moving at all. But then, "Even if we couldn't stop the end from coming, at least we'd be in it together. It's hard, being all by myself in it, being the only one who knows what's all going on. I feel . . ."

"Lonely?" we offer.

"Yeah. Real lonely."

"It's hard when our loved ones don't believe us. But this time loop has actually given us a shittily wrapped gift, Gabbro. You know that your friends don't believe you, which means that you can save yourself precious minutes trying to convince them of something they are unready or unwilling to hear. You can use this time to just tell them how much you love them, and miss them, and engage in community with the moments you have."

"Hmm, it would be nice to reminisce with Hornfels. Could even try to radio over to Esker. I know they get lonely out there on the Lunar Outpost. Hearthians haven't had much use for that post in years, but Esker just likes the routine of it, I think—even if it's lonely sometimes."

"Yes, that sounds like a great idea. You can spend time reminiscing and helping others feel less lonely too."

"I still wish there was something I could do about the end."

"Of course you do. To quote a famous philosopher, 'So do all who live to see such times. But that is not for them to decide. All we have to decide is what to do with the time that is given us.' And that's all you can do, Gabbro. That's what we call radical acceptance. We accept that things are as they are and stop fighting their inevitability."

"I guess if I accept that I can't stop the time loop on my own it frees up some energetic space. And I could still mention it to Hornfels from time to time." Gabbro laughs.

"You did a time joke."

"Yeah, I did. Laughing feels nice. Haven't laughed in several loops at least. Yeah, I can keep mentioning it, but maybe with less expectation attached to it. That way I'm giving Hornfels the option to hear me out while not feeling like it's all on me."

"That sounds like a great idea, Gabbro. You're starting to embrace the idea of nonattachment. It will help you to move through this experience with a bit more space."

"Ha! You made a space joke!"

"We sure did." We chuckle with them.

"Well, our time's almost up, friends."

"Would you like us to loop back with you? We could certainly talk more if that would help."

"You know, I think I've got this. At least, I'd want to try out what we've talked about on my own for a while. If this loop is still going in a day or two in your time, maybe check back in with me?"

"We can certainly do that, Gabbro." We hesitate, our hands hovering over our call buttons.

"You worried about me? Well, that's fair. I'm worried about me too. But worry is not such a bad thing. Sometimes it just means a thing is important. The trick is to be with what's important right now. And I've got some tools to try that out. So thank you."

"Any time, Gabbro."

"Ha! Another time joke. I really like you two. Shame we don't have more time. But I suppose we always want more time."

"That's very wise, Gabbro."

Gabbro shrugs, as the world around them begins to fade. "Pain can make us wise, if you let it. See you out there."

The oceans rise around us as Gabbro blurs from vision. We blink our eyes and find our virtual selves have returned. We're back in our offices, and the sun is bright outside.

FANFIC CASE STUDY QUESTIONS:
It's That Time Again for a Few Questions!

- If you've played *Outer Wilds*, what was your first reaction when you learned that your avatar only had twenty-two minutes to live during each play through? If you have yet to play the game, use what you've learned from the case study to describe the feelings that came up for you when you learned that Gabbro has been living and dying on repeat.
- What do you think of Gabbro's new nonattachment to outcomes?
- What do you think motivates the protagonist to keep living life, albeit on a twenty-two-minute repeating loop?

MINDFUL MEDITATION:
Noticing the Change in Every Breath

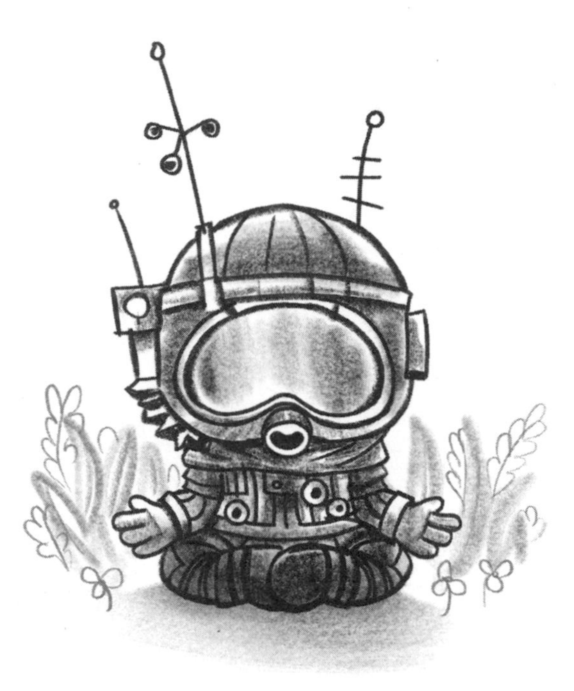

Find a comfortable space where you can relax for a few minutes. Consider reclining if that will help you relax without focusing on any bodily discomfort that you might be experiencing. Once you've found a comfortable space, give yourself permission to just relax. Feel free to close your eyes, find a gazing object, or simply soften your gaze. Start to bring your awareness to your breath. Notice what the air feels like as it comes in and goes out. Notice the texture of the air, the temperature on both the inhale and exhale. Feel where in your body the breath originates. Is it in your chest? Or does it originate deep in your belly? No matter what you find, allow it to be simply information. If you find that you would like to make a change to the way that you are breathing, give yourself permission to try that out, and know that you can always come back to the way things were. No decision here is final.

Notice how the breath influences the way you feel in your body. Do you feel more energized or calmed? Do you notice any particular sensations in your body as the air moves? Again, assigning no judgment to what you find; this is simply information. Every few breaths, check back in with all of these areas again. Notice how the breath feels, where it comes from in the body, and how it influences your body. Your breath is changeable. It isn't the same from moment to moment and day to day, and that's just fine. Our circumstances are constantly changing. We cannot catch a breath and hold it in a jar; it lives by moving, and so do we. We invite you to practice the acceptance of change just as you practice the acceptance of your changing breath as you move through your day.

Now What? Living in a Rewritten Story

No doubt—endings are hard. But then again . . .
nothing ever really ends, does it?

—CHUCK, AKA GOD, IN *SUPERNATURAL*, "SWAN SONG"[277]

You've done it! You've reached the end of this book; or very nearly the end. You've learned how to sit with intense emotions, accept the realities of a struggling planet, and, by so doing, provide aid where and how you can. You've learned how to care for your anxiety gremlins and depression Demogorgon, use the Westworld Construct to challenge the status quo, take back your story, and rewrite your life. In the words of Hagrid, "Harry—Yer a wizard."[278] That is, you're a hero. But you knew that all along, didn't you?

We have just a few tools left to teach before we depart as your stalwart guides. Before we begin, we remind you as always to take what works and leave the rest. As the writer of your own Therapeutic Fanfiction, you are in a position to know best what you do and don't need. And, when you're not sure, you can always turn to chapter 10 to find a trained healer to ask for help. As our favorite problematic headmaster says, "You will . . . find that help will always be given at Hogwarts to those who ask for it."[279]

Throughout this book, we've invited you to journal either literally or mentally. As you read this final chapter, you might find it helpful to have those musings handy. The act of writing and reflecting on this book has been you answering the call to adventure. You've already started to create change in your life. As you continue your quest beyond these pages, remember that you can always come back to consult this text anew. The hero's journey is cyclical because, as Q says to Picard, "The trial never ends."[280] The trial to which Q is referring is life itself.

We hope that reading and reflecting on this book are both an end and a beginning as you start to integrate the tools of Therapeutic Fanfiction into your life. First and foremost, this is about honoring your fandom attachments. Whether it's your love for Madden NFL, Max Payne, Jane Austen, Dean Winchester, or Arya Stark, these attachments are real and profound. And these feelings help you to know what stories and characters you need and when. If you're looking to continue therapeutic fanficcing a challenging relationship with your family of origin, Dean or Sam Winchester might be your hunters. But, if you're looking to navigate the hellscape that is online dating, Jane Austen has some tips and tricks for you. Therapeutic Fanfiction is where whimsy meets analysis.

Therapeutic Fanfic: 2 Fic 2 Furious

We've reached the end of our road together, and now we are but two cars idling side by side. Before we go, let's recap what we've learned in a list.

Therapeutic Fanfic Step by Step

1. Gather Your Fellowship: Both IRL and Fandom Attachments
2. Question Your Questing: Discover What Your Quest Is About
3. Pairing Up: Match Your Struggles to the Helpers on Your Quest
4. Gather Any Additional Tools:
    A. Westworld Construct
    B. Crossing Guard
    C. Externalizing the Problem

    D. Personification
    E. Fandom Attachments
    F. Totem
    G. Posttraumatic growth
    H. Resilience
    I. Rules, Roles, and Boundaries, aka the Stardew Valley House
    J. Hunters' Journal
    K. Trust Staircase
    L. Stress Mountain
    M. Introvert-Extrovert Spectrum
5. Rewrite Your Story
    A. Explore and/or Make Some Meaning
    B. Keep Your Meaning Close with a Totem

Take a moment and look over the work you have already done in your journaling or all around your mind palace. Consider how you feel toward these ideas now that you've had more time to reflect. Without assigning any judgment, just notice. Are there any changes that you'd like to make? You get to make changes as frequently or as infrequently as you'd like. This is your story.

If you're just starting out on your Therapeutic Fanfiction journey, the easiest place to begin is with steps one and two. Make a list of the most resonant fandom characters to you, and start to bring this list into your daily life. Perhaps in the morning while making your first beverage of the day, you pause and ask yourself, *How would Agent Dale Cooper start his morning?*[281] He'd make a hot cuppa Joe and have a donut, for which he'd make no apologies. As Coop says, "Every day, once a day, give yourself a present." Take some time while you prepare your beverage to playfully engage with the image of Coop while you complete your morning routine. Trying out being with different fandom attachments throughout your day will help you get a sense of who might be most helpful in a specific circumstance. Consider this same example but with a character such as Hagrid. Mornings with Hagrid might not feel as relaxed. He's likely out feeding Buckbeak, a feral half horse half eagle, and getting snorted at; he's perhaps not the best morning companion.[282] But you need to try out different companions before you can figure out who's the best fit. Which fandom attachments allow you to feel like you're being seen and that you aren't alone? Which fandom attachments provide you support when you need it? Start to identify which folks add important aspects to your life when you need them.

If you're at a spot where you're feeling practiced in matching fandom attachments to challenging situations, then you're in a middle place—a medium place, to be exact. When feelings are neutral to positive, you're able to readily call up Samwise when you need support, Storm when you need encouragement, and Thor's hammer when you need to reground in your personal truth. But you need some practice in knowing whom to call on during periods of stress and struggle. This is an opportunity to find ways to remind yourself of who has helped in the past and to give yourself cues to call upon them, perhaps with a mighty and heroic post-it note on your computer keyboard that reads "Mjolnir!" so that you never forget to call for your enchanted hammer.[283] Some other ways that heroes have found work for them to remember these ideas are through enchantments on their mobile devices or putting memories in a pensieve. We encourage you to use whatever means helps you to call upon the mythic power you need.

If you're already comfortable calling on specific characters or fandom tools for help during times of strife, then you might be ready for some more complex Therapeutic Fanfiction: time for some existential dread. You are ready to ask the big questions: Why am I here? What does all this mean? I know that I matter but in what way? Stories and play are how early human beings first learned how to ask these questions and explored ways to answer them. The power of myth is still here for us, and, when mindfully deployed, it can change your life and the lives of your community. Recall chapter 2 and chapter 11 and the idea that every rock has ripples. You are the rock.[cxv]

Joseph Campbell had some serious thoughts about the power of stories and, more specifically, about the powers that they awaken within us.[284] A story is a powerful tool, but it isn't the agent of change, nor is it the hero you seek. No, reader, you are. So if symbolically holding Mjolnir allows you to feel the power of Thor, you are the one holding the power, not the story of

[cxv] Well, not "The Rock." But you know what we mean.

Thor. Does this mean you can literally shoot lightning from your fists? No, probably not. But it does mean that you can create powerful connections with your physical body. If this resonates with you, it likely holds a key to the way you make meaning. Fundamentally, life is about connecting with other life. Perhaps you connect best by reaching out to offer a consensual handshake or offer an affirming hug. Neuroscience shows the power and necessity for consensual physical touch among human beings and other creatures.[285] Owning your internal Mjolnir power, the power that you feel from physical connection, can help you to decide what is meaningful to you. If you feel strong with a Mjolnir in your hands, perhaps you also feel strong when you pet a kitten or make a delicious sandwich for your roommate. These can also help you feel the power of a Viking god. No matter where you're at on this journey, you now have the tools and guides to help you begin or continue on this journey of change and self-discovery. Go forth, hero!

How to Share Your Story

Perhaps you've already been engaging with the people in your life about what you've learned in this book, or perhaps you've been waiting until you finished to bring this up to the people around you. Whatever choice you've made, we support you. We'd like to let you know about some potential stumbling blocks that folks sometimes have when they begin a newly written story. Some folks around you, remember, are still living in their old Westworld Construct, and when something comes along to challenge that narrative, they can get nervous or defensive. The desire for the status quo to remain, well, quo is so strong that folks will often fight against change, even if someone else is the one making the change.

We invite you to have some compassion for the folks around you. You can relate to what they're going through, since you probably felt some similar feelings when you first picked up this book. They might also be grieving the loss of the way you were; even though you're feeling really great about your new story, they might miss the old story and that's understandable. Try to practice your skills to continue to find compassion for others and for yourself.

How do you decide to whom you want to share your story? You may want to use the tool you learned in chapter 7 known as the trust staircase. You may want to write in your journal, or reflect in your mind palace, in order to come up with a list of folks with whom you want to share this new story. Now comes the challenging part. What feelings arise when you conjure up each person in this list—love, hope, fear, pain, sadness, joy, comfort, regret, anger? For folks who trigger feelings of fear, sadness, or anger, you might want to hold off on sharing until you've practiced sharing with folks who feel safer. People who evoke fear, sadness, or anger may have hurt you in the past. So you want to feel practiced and ready before you try to walk up the trust staircase with them. When we share our story, we give folks the opportunity to show us whether or not we can continue to move up the staircase with them. If folks have a big negative reaction, that might mean that it's time to stay on the stair you're currently on or move down a step until they're able to hold space for this new information.

To help you begin this dialogue with trusted friends and/or family, we've included a letter template, conversation example, and a book-jacket blurb below.

Letter Template

Dear Hagrid,

I'm writing this note to tell you a little bit about the journey I've been on. It's been both an external and internal quest, and in the process I've changed. Some of these changes were planned out by me and my helper/guide/therapist. Here are a few examples of some mindful changes I have made in my life and am working on maintaining: ____________________

____.

You are an important person to me, and I wanted to let you know about these changes so that you'll understand if I seem different. If I don't seem different, that's OK too. I hope that if you have questions about the changes I've made or have thoughts about these changes, you'll reach out and communicate them to me with compassion. I really appreciate/feel grateful to you for ____.

Looking forward to seeing you soon,

Harry

Conversation Template

Before I read this book, I felt _______, __________, and ___________. Some things had happened to me that were really hard. And while I did my best to cope with them, when I look back on it now, some of my coping strategies caused some problems. [Optionally, you could explain what some of these problems were.]

During the process of reading this book, I learned many things about myself and the world around me. For example, I learned that fandom attachments are real and important. I hope that you will be open to hearing more about my fandom friends because they are really important to me, just like you. I also learned ____

____.

This process has changed parts of me. An example of something that has changed is my ability to sit with big or intense feelings. The tools of personification and externalization help me see the ways that I am connected to my feelings but not equivalent to my feelings. Because of this change, I want to share my feelings with you more often. And I want to hear about your feelings too. I understand that this is different. How do you feel about this difference? Another example of something that has changed is ______

____.

I worked very hard to rewrite the story of my life. I recognize that it might feel strange and that I might seem different. And I understand that it might take you a while to get to know this new story. I will do my best to give you the space to do that. I just want you to know how much different I feel with my story. I would describe myself now as feeling _____________. I'm looking forward to continuing to share my story with you.

Book Jacket Template

[Name your story. Be as flashy or not as you want.]

In a world where society says you should [a previously held Westworld Construct], one person dared to resist the status quo. [Your name] embarked on an epic emotional journey with the crew of the Starship Therapise. [Your name] faced many hard truths, such as [something difficult you faced] but also found [some things you're proud of] along the way. [Your name] rewrote [your pronoun] story and gets to live a more authentic life. In the end, [your name] learned [something you learned about yourself] about [your pronoun] and became [your pronoun] own hero!

—

Once you've shared your new story, a dialogue has begun. Or put another way, you and the other person are beginning a co-hero's journey that will hopefully lead to increased mutual understanding, compassion, and affection. Just like in your personal hero's journey, there will be challenges along the way. You may even need to get some support from a trusted mentor or find a therapist—either a couple or family therapist.

Hero's Journey Redux

Like Aughra of *The Dark Crystal* series[286] and movie once said, "Endings, beginnings—all the same."[287] Very much in keeping with Aughra's wisdom, we invite you to recall chapter 1 and our first discussion around the hero's journey, that ancient myth or "first story" present in all cultures, regions, and countries. It is a story that resonates across the human conception of time and space because it tells the story of each of us. It is the story of you.

Below, you'll find an interactive case study that will help you as you continue your own hero's journey. We invite you to refer to your notes—either literal or in your virtual mind palace—as you start to draft the story of your hero's journey. This is a cyclical process; we invite you to revisit, re-create, and renew your quest as often as you need. In the spirit of fandom attachment—and what would we be without these precious and playful connections—we invite you to take us with you.

CASE STUDY:
You, the Hero

We are working in our offices on the Starship Therapise and receive a hail from the universe. It is you! You need our services, and, friend, we are here for you. Please join us in our offices, with or without a cup of tea, and let's get to work.

"Welcome, please take a seat. It's so lovely to finally meet you in person! What brings you in to see us?"

You pause and then begin to tell us the story of what brought you to this point in your journey: "_______________________________________"

"Fascinating. It sounds like you've been through a lot. So you picked up our book. Thank you for that. What's been helpful so far?"

You carefully consider this question as you reflect on some of the things that you've learned while reading this book. We notice that you seem deep in thought and ask, "Would you like to share some of your reflections with us? Anything that stood out to you during this journey we've been on together?"

You look up and say, "_______________________________________"

"Thank you so much for sharing that. It's amazing how we can start to see things differently, isn't it? How are you feeling about your story now that you've started to rewrite it?"

"_______________________________________"

"Who are some of the fandom mentors or guides that supported you along this journey?"

"_______________________________________"

"Great choices! What are the aspects of those folks that speak to your values? What brought you to decide on them over others?"

"_______________________________________"

"We've got to say that you have some amazing insights. It's so brave to look inside ourselves like this. What are some of the challenges that you might face in your life beyond these pages, and how might the tools you've learned help you?"

"_______________________________________"

"Of course, that makes sense. You've done so much work, and of course there's more to do, but you've got this. What else would you like us to know before we close out?"

"____"

"It has been an honor to serve with you on the Starship Therapise. You are always welcome to return whenever you need. Live long and prosper."

YOGA MASTER PRACTICE:
Revisiting What You Have Learned and Putting It All Together

GRAB YOUR GREMLINS

1. Mountain Pose

   Begin in a comfortable standing or seated position with your arms at your sides. Take a moment to simply observe the gremlins that are crawling around.

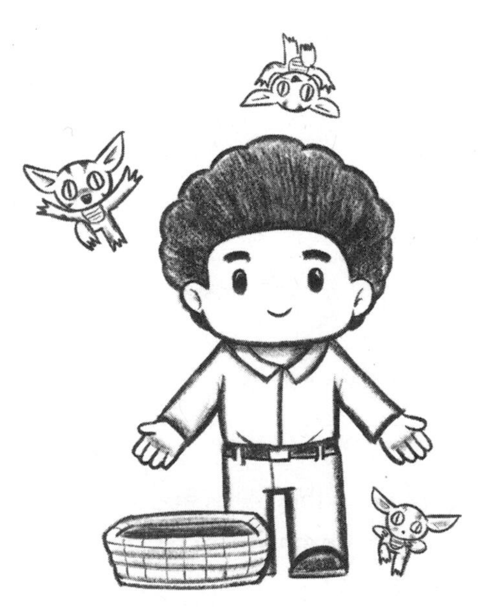

2. Upward Salute

Identify a particularly troublesome gremlin, and reach up high to grab it.

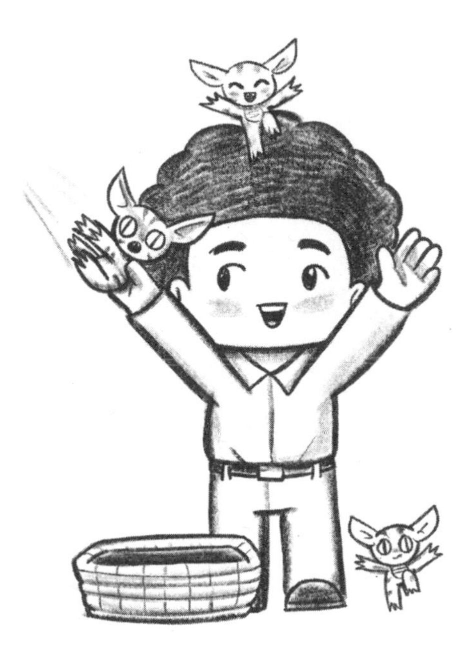

3. Standing Forward Bend

Fold the upper body forward, and place the gremlin in its basket.

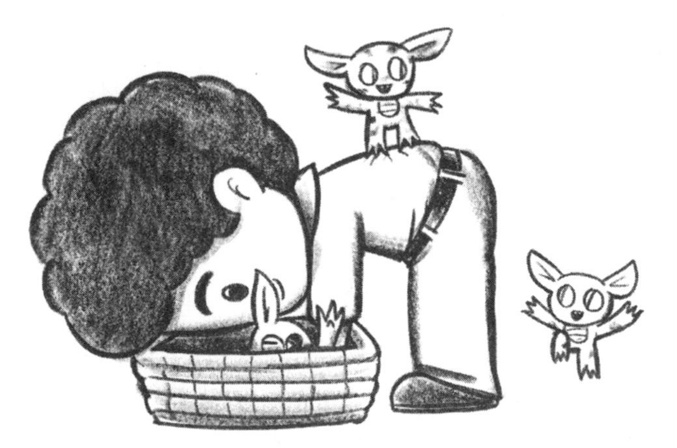

4. Halfway Lift

It will naturally crawl right out, so lift your upper body halfway to catch the little rascal.

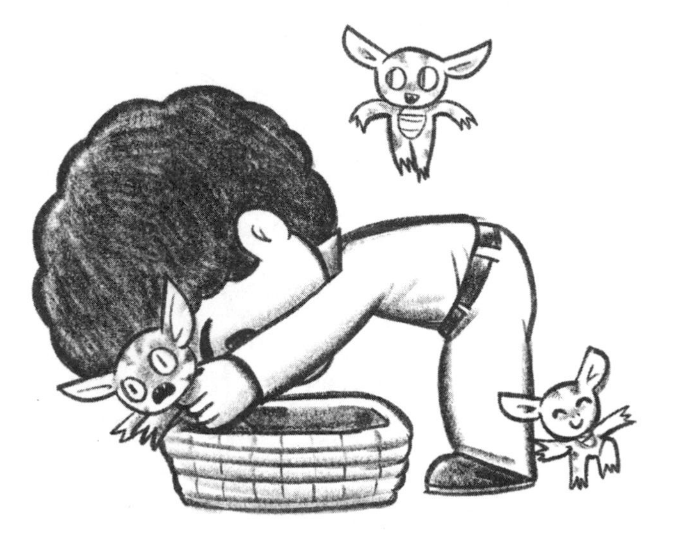

5. Standing Forward Bend

Fold forward again to place the gremlin in its basket.

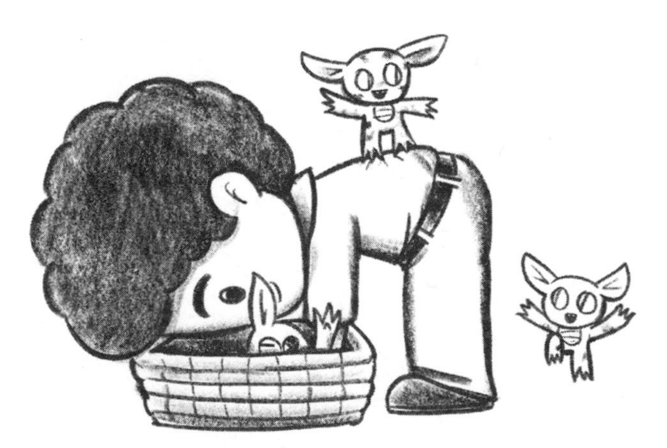

6. Upward Salute

   Reach arms high up overhead again, and repeat for all other gremlins that you find.

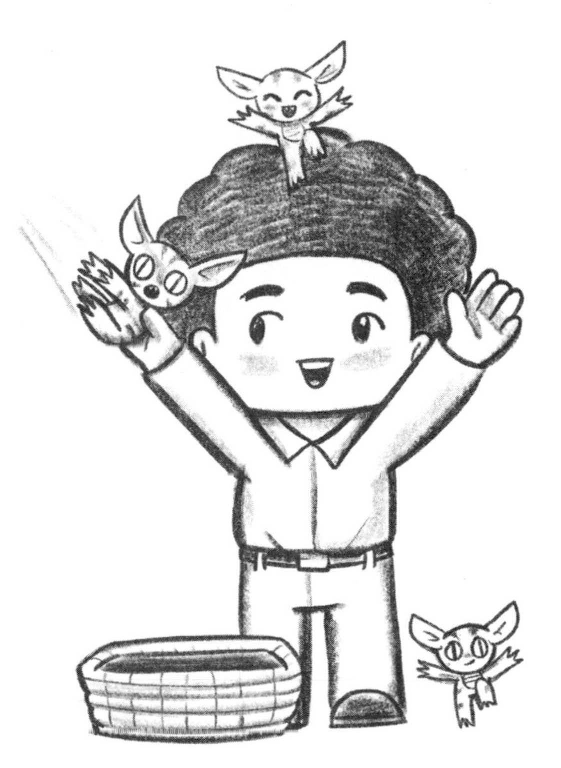

7. Hands to Heart Center

   Once you are out of gremlins, bring your hands to your heart, and allow yourself to feel gratitude for the work that you've done.

PREPARE FOR THE BOSS BATTLE

8. Seated or Standing Mountain Pose

   Picture yourself just about to fight the big boss. Notice the feelings as they start to rise in your body.

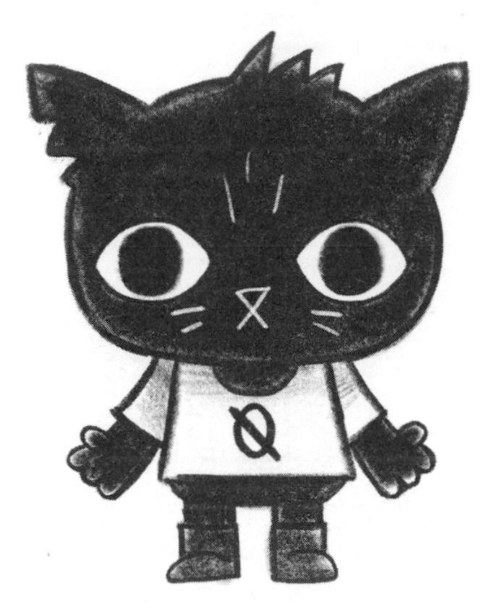

9. Backbend Pose

As the feelings rise up, lift your arms up to the sky. Picture yourself having just defeated your foe. Celebrate this accomplishment by taking a baby backbend and sending out a thank you from your heart. Bring your arms back upward and then down to your heart. Imagine a protective shield around yourself.

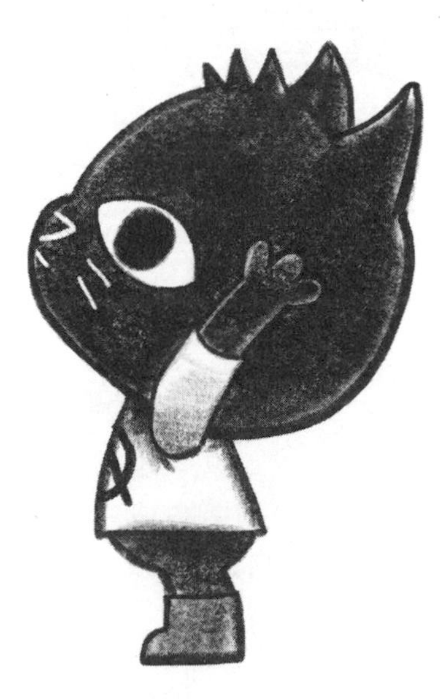

10. Side Stretch Pose

Explore the edges of your protective shield by moving from right to left, back and forward a few times. If interlacing your fingers is uncomfortable for any reason, keep your arms wide.

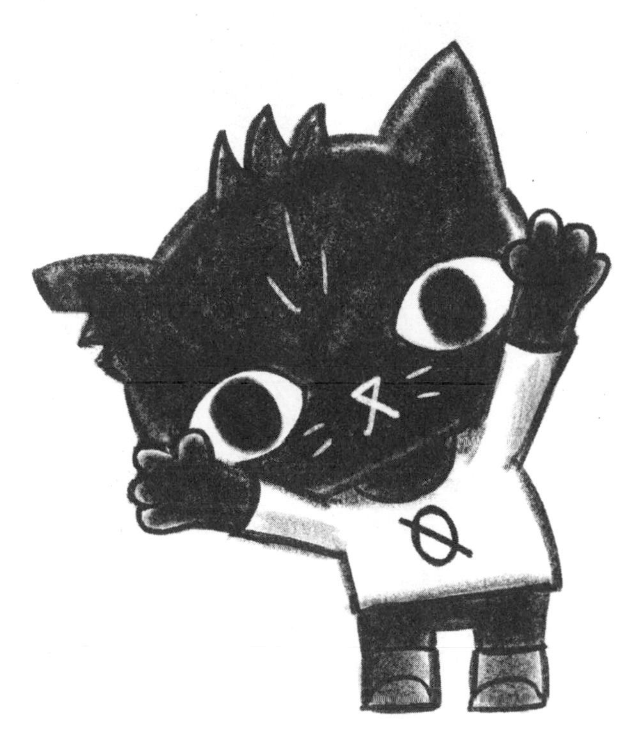

11. Crescent Lunge Pose

Now step one foot forward. You can stay here if that's comfortable, or you can bend your front knee and come up onto the ball mount of your back foot. You can also drop to your back knee. Picture yourself striding to victory. If it helps, you can even move your arms as if you are walking toward your destiny. Hold for five to ten breaths, and then switch sides. Get ready to win.

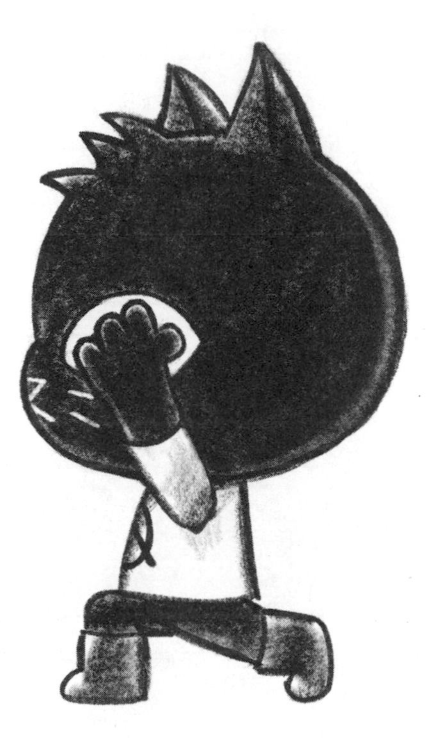

12. Seated or Standing Mountain Pose

Return to your starting pose, and return your awareness to your breath. With each inhale, think, *I am,* and with each exhale, *a hero.* Remember this mantra for when you return to the game or any big boss battles that you face.

STAY STRONG

13. You Are the Sword

Begin standing or seated in a chair, with feet a comfortable distance apart and hands at your sides.

A. Pause here for a moment, noticing the feel of your feet connected with the earth, your shoulders broad and confident.

B. Imagine that you have a sword in your hand but that even if you didn't it wouldn't matter. You *are* the sword. With every inhale, think, *I am*, and with every exhale, *the sword*. Continue this for three to five breaths.

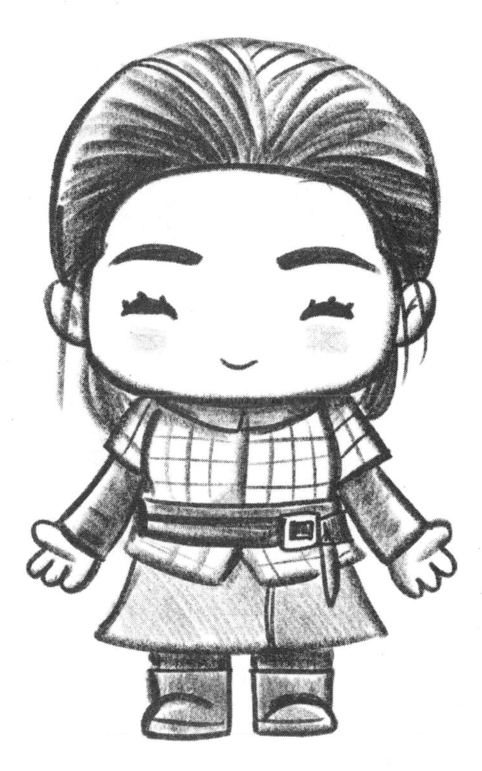

14. Fighting Stance

Take a wide stance with your feet.

A. Turn both feet outward; then turn both feet inward. Finally turn your right foot out, and leave your left foot turned inward. Bend your right knee. Be mindful to keep your knee above or behind your ankle. Water dancers must protect their valuable knees. Bring your arms out to shoulder height, and grasp your imaginary sword.

B. Pause here for a moment, and feel your feet grounded to the floor and your head lifted toward the ceiling. You are both solid and quick-footed.

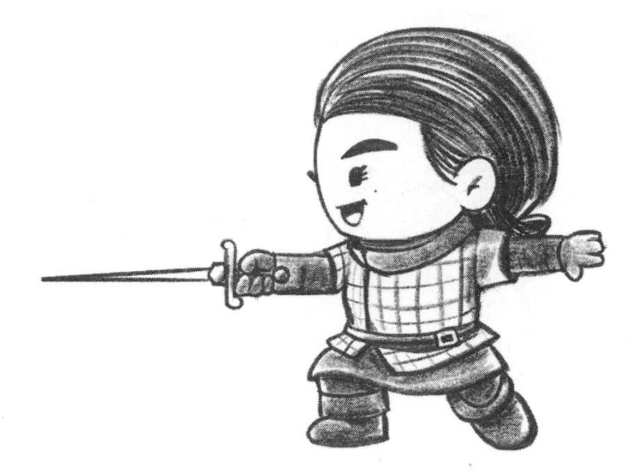

15. Forward Thrust

Thrust your right arm with your "sword" forward toward your imaginary opponent while keeping your feet flat on the floor. You are both grounded and agile.

16. Downward Thrust

Your forward thrust does not collide with your opponent, so you try again by sweeping your right arm down as your left arm reaches high.

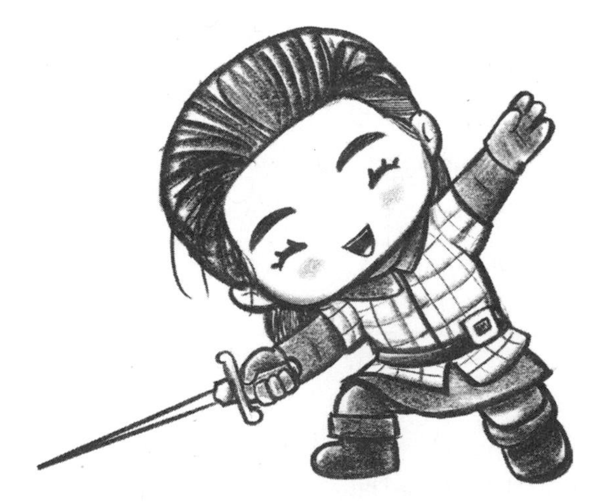

17. Upward Thrust

    Once more you show your strength by sweeping your right arm all the way up to the sky while your left arm comes down your left leg. You have made your mark on your opponent, who retreats, giving you time to return to your fighting stance.

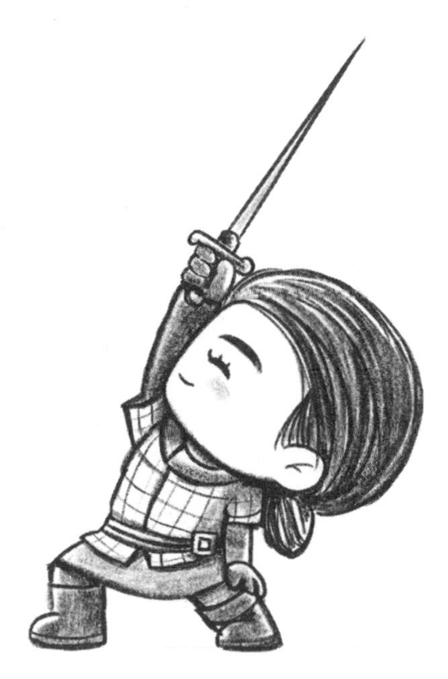

18. Return to the Fight

    Straighten your right knee, turning your right foot in and your left foot out and bending your left knee. Jauntily toss your sword from your right hand to your left, and begin your water dance on the other side.

19. Not Today

    Once you have moved through the dance as many times as suits you, use a heel-and-toe motion to get your feet back to your comfortable stance of the Sword Pose. Return your hands to your sides, or, if it feels best, bring your palms to touch in front of your chest. Repeat your mantra, "I am the sword."

FINDING BALANCE

20. Great Deku or Tree Pose

A. Begin with your feet a comfortable distance apart and your arms at your sides.

B. Shift weight onto your left foot, and turn your right knee outward. Feel free to leave your right toe on the floor or have your right heel pressed against your left ankle. As you feel more balanced, you can move your right foot up your left leg as high as is comfortable. (Just avoid your knee joint; your knee will thank you.)

C. Your arms can be wherever you prefer: on your hips, up overhead like a tree, or resting on a chair or the wall for balance. Once you find your balance, try to hold it for three to five full breaths, and then release. Switch sides, and repeat.

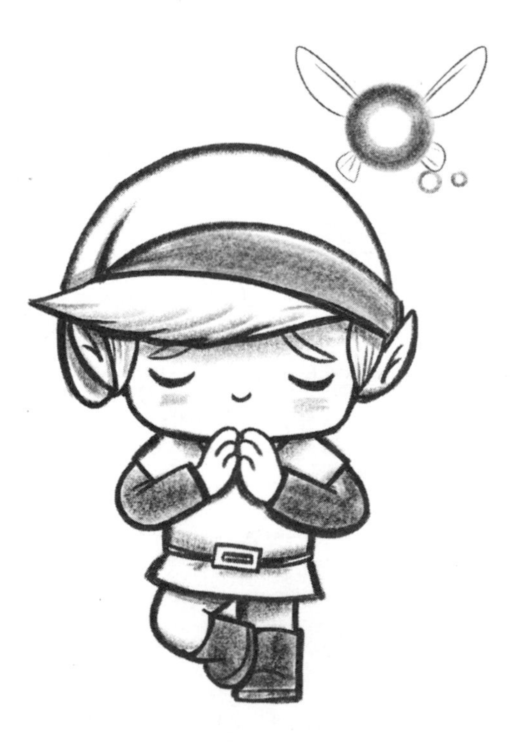

21. Rito or Eagle Pose

A. Begin with your feet a comfortable distance apart and your arms at your sides.

B. Lift arms up overhead, and identify your right hand (hey!).

C. Bring your right arm under your left, giving yourself a hug.

If you find that you want more stretch and the option is available to you, you can cross your arms at both your elbows and your wrists.

D. Now sit way back in an imaginary chair (we know).

You're welcome to stay right here; it's a perfectly good spot to be or . . .

Shift your weight onto your left foot, and bring your right leg up and over the left.

E. Some folks like to cross first and then sit back; some cross just at the ankle. The fun is that you get to make this pose your own!

F. Once you find your balance, see if you can hold it for three to five breaths, and then release. Next, try on the other side!

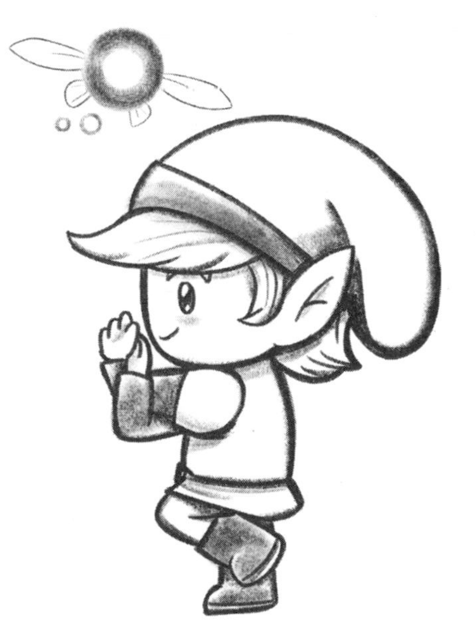

22. Link in Flight or Airplane Pose

A. Begin with your feet a comfortable distance apart and your arms at your sides.

B. Step your right foot forward.

Feel free to keep your left toes on the ground, or you can begin to lift that leg as far as comfortable, but be mindful not to tip your upper body too far forward, or your Link might crash-land.

C. Sweep both arms back behind you.

D. Lift your chest like a proud Link.

E. Balance here for three to five breaths, and feel the Breath of the Wild in your hair. Then release, and repeat while switching sides.

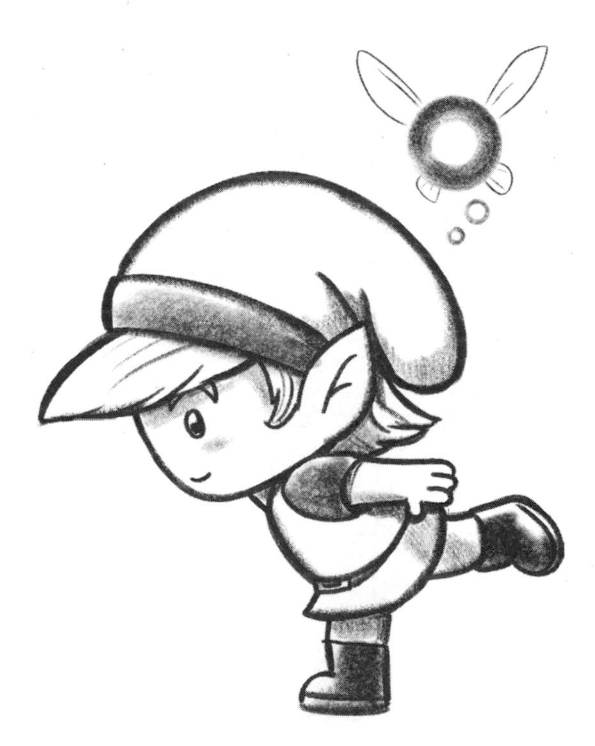

MAKE SOME MAGIC

23. Heart Pose

Bring your hands together, palms touching with your thumbs touching the center of your sternum. This position will be where the spells begin and end, and you will return to it between each of the other poses.

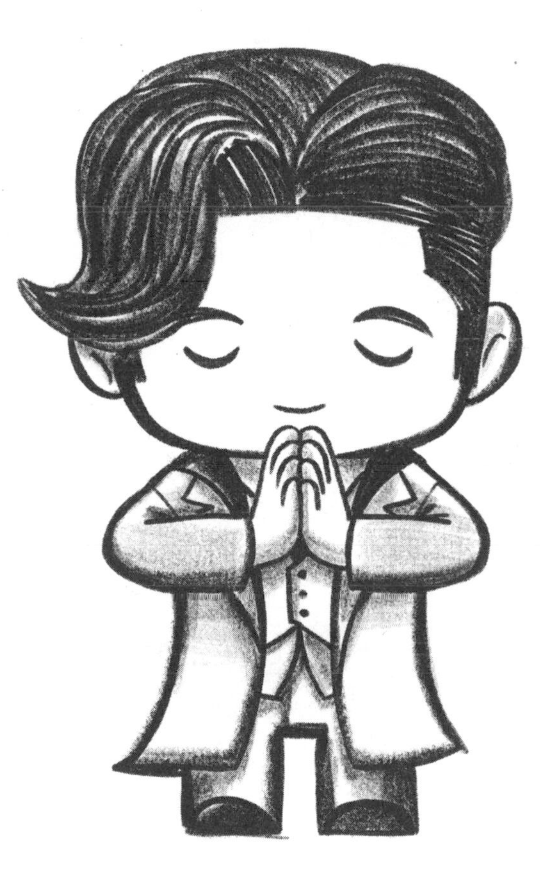

24. Removing Wards Pose

Starting from Heart Pose, twist your hands so that your fingers face your opposite wrists. Slide your fingers so that you can clasp them together with your opposite hand. Clasp them tightly.

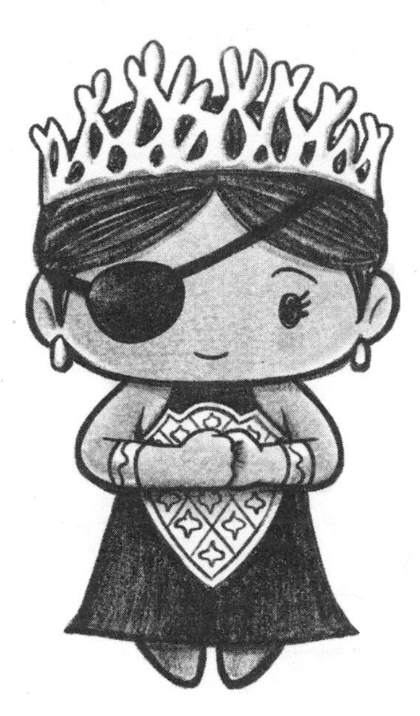

25. Return to your Heart Pose.

26. High King Margo Pose

From Heart Pose, interlace all ten fingers, and then release your index finger, creating a steeple grip. Point your steeple forward with conviction.

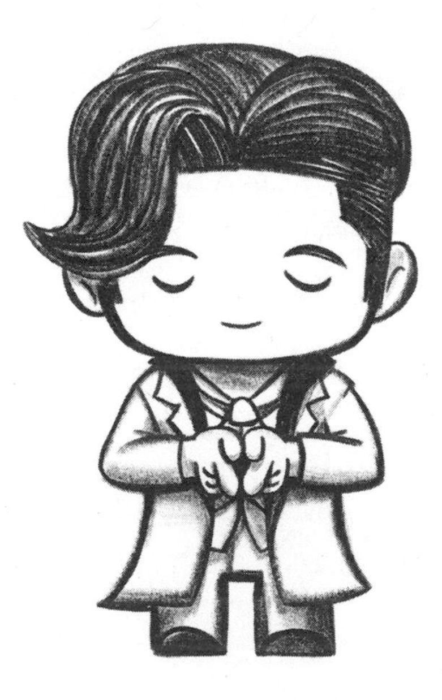

27. Return to your Heart Pose.

28. Fillorian Sage Pose

Place the back of your right hand on top of your left palm, and touch your thumbs together. Pause here, and allow the Fillorian sages to calm you.

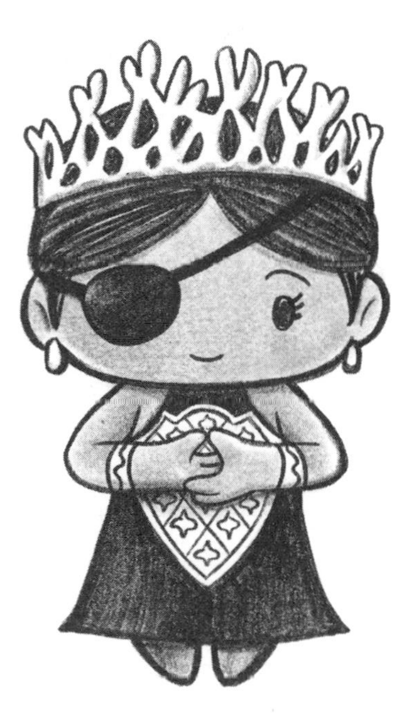

29. Return to your Heart Pose.

30. High King Eliot Pose

With the elegance of Eliot, bring your hands in front of you at about shoulder height, palms facing forward. Bring your index and ring finger to touch your thumb on each hand.

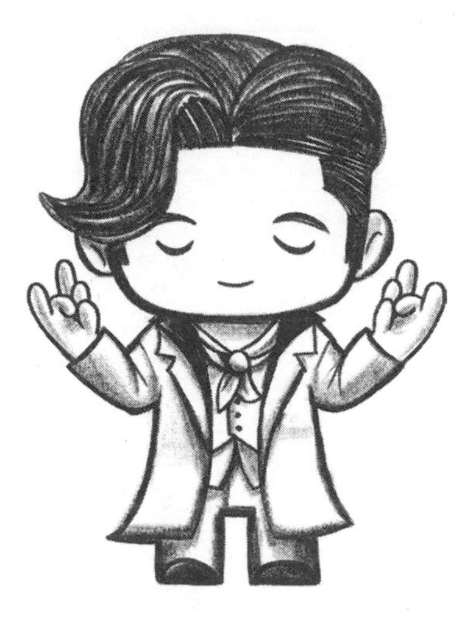

31. Return to your Heart Pose.

32. Unshakable Trust Pose

From your Heart Pose, interlace your fingers and release your thumbs. With the ferocity that only Margo can bring, forcefully press the backs of your hands forward.

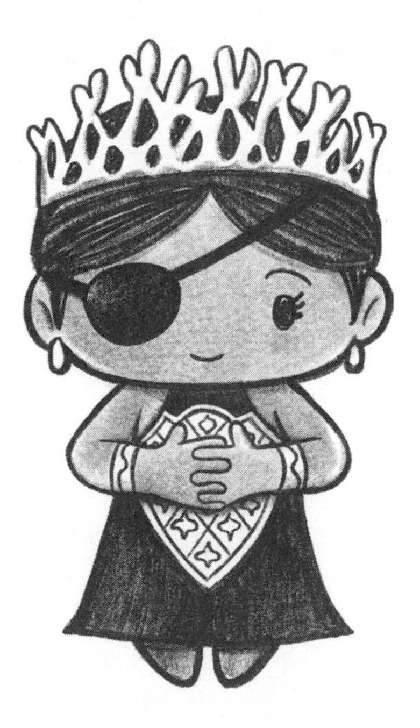

33. Return to your Heart Pose.

Spend a few moments here in your Heart Pose, and offer yourself both gratitude and compassion. This was an incredible journey. You've accomplished so much. And, yet, you've only just begun.

Fandom Mandala Coloring Sheet: An Opportunity for Quiet Reflection on the Journey

At last, reader, we come to the end. But harkening back to Chuck's quote at the beginning of this chapter, nothing ever really ends because our journey is circular—starting and ending and starting again. We have included this mandala for your quiet reflection.[cxvi] It has been an honor to serve with you on the Starship Therapise. May you live long and prosper.

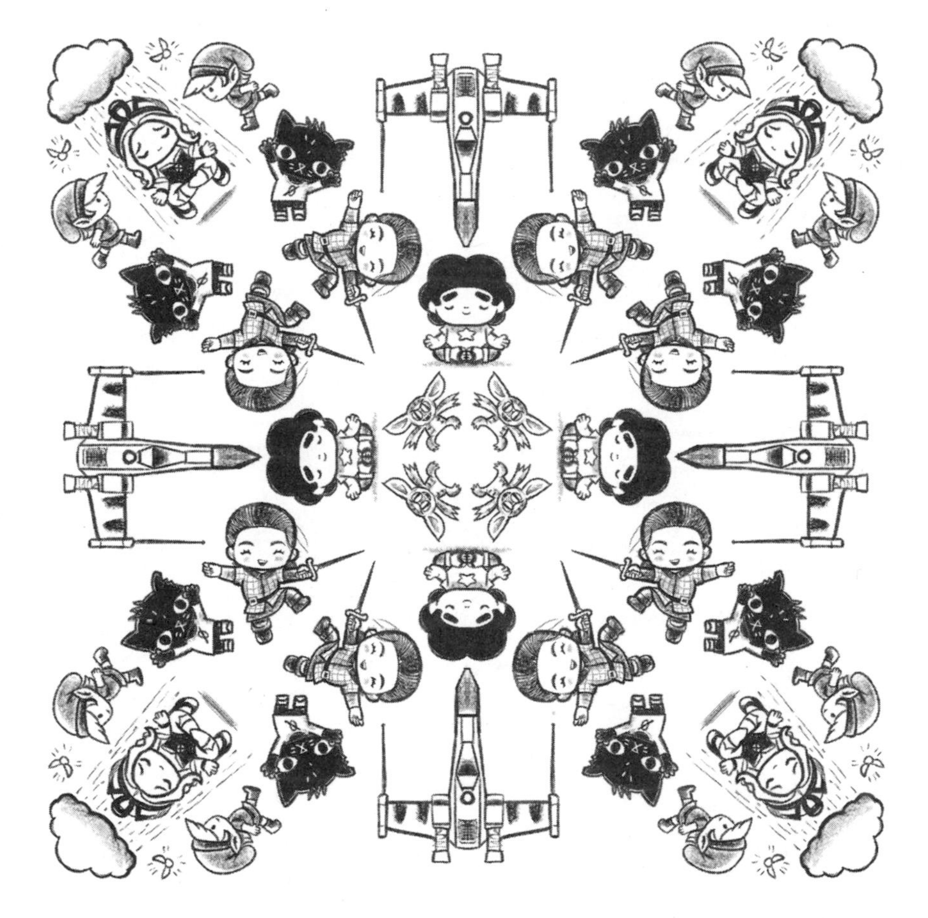

[cxvi] With crayons! Or colored pencils! (You get the idea.)

RESOURCES

Mind

Aesthetics and Politics by Theodor Adorna, Walter Benjamin, Ernst Bloch, Bertolt Brecht, & Georg Lukács

The Hero with a Thousand Faces by Joseph Campbell

The Collected Works of C. G. Jung: The Archetypes and the Collective Unconscious by C. G. Jung

Black Skin, White Masks by Frantz Fanon

Seeing Race Again: Countering Colorblindness across the Disciplines, edited by Kimberlé Williams Crenshaw, Luke Charles Harris, Daniel Martinez HoSang, & George Lipsitz

My Grandmother's Hands by Resmaa Menakem

Body

The Body Keeps the Score by Bessel van der Kolk

Body Respect: What Conventional Health Books Get Wrong, Leave Out, and Just Plain Fail to Understand about Weight by Linda Bacon & Lucy Aphramor

The Body Is Not an Apology: The Power of Radical Self-Love by Sonya Renee Taylor

The Diet Survivor's Handbook: 60 Lessons in Eating, Acceptance and Self-Care by Judith Matz & Ellen Frankel

Star Trek: Body by Starfleet: A Fitness Guide by Robb Pearlman

Yoga Where You Are: Customize Your Practice for Your Body and Your Life by Dianne Bondy & Kat Heagberg

Fandom

Using Superheroes and Villains in Counseling and Play Therapy, edited by Lawrence Rubin, PhD

Superhero Therapy: Mindfulness Skills to Help Teens and Young Adults Deal with Anxiety, Depression, and Trauma by Janina Scarlet, PhD

The Fanfiction Reader: Folktales for a Digital Age by Francesca Coppa
Black Panther Psychology: Hidden Kingdoms, edited by Travis Langley, PhD, & Alex Simmons
The Psychology of Zelda: Linking Our World to the Legend of Zelda Series, edited by Anthony Bean, PhD
Supernatural Psychology: Roads Less Traveled, edited by Travis Langley, PhD, & Lynn S. Zubernis, PhD

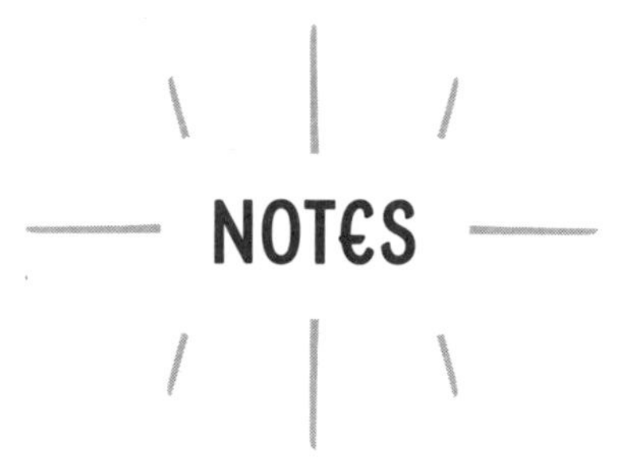

NOTES

Introduction

[1] Braga, et al. (1994, May 23).

Chapter 1

[2] Bioware (2012).
[3] Roddenberry (1966–1969).
[4] Bacon-Smith (1992); Jenkins (2013).
[5] Coppa (2017).
[6] Ker (1993); Van der Veer (2011).
[7] Ker (1993).
[8] Jung (1990a); Jung (2009).
[9] Akinyela (2002).
[10] Berger & Luckmann (1966); Freedman & Combs (1996).
[11] Ker (1993).
[12] Fanon (2008).
[13] Fanon (2005).
[14] Jung (1990a).
[15] Campbell (1949/2008).
[16] Campbell (1949/2008).
[17] Bioware (2007); Bioware (2010); Bioware (2012).
[18] Campbell (1949/2008).
[19] White & Epston (1990/2015).
[20] White (2007), p. 26.
[21] White & Epston (1990/2015).
[22] White (2007).
[23] Gardner & Knowles (2008).
[24] Maggs (2015).
[25] Horton & Wohl (1956); Eyal & Dailey (2012).
[26] Garski & Mastin (2020).

[27] Cole & Leets (1999).
[28] van der Kolk, (2014/2015), pp. 58–59.
[29] Cohen (2010).
[30] Whedon, et al. (1997–2003).
[31] *Buffy the Vampire Slayer Season Eight* (2007–2011).
[32] Benioff, et al. (2011–2019).

Chapter 2

[33] Pitts, et al. (March 22, 2020).
[34] Freedman & Combs (1996).
[35] Abrams, et al. (2016–present).
[36] Berger & Luckmann (1966).
[37] Wachowski & Wachowski (1999).
[38] Minuchin & Fishman (1981); Whitaker (1982).
[39] Nintendo (1992).
[40] Dolynski & Alexander (November 22, 1968).
[41] Matz & Frankel (2004/2014).
[42] Matz & Frankel (2004/2014).
[43] Bacon & Aphramor (2011).
[44] *Bitch Planet,* #1 (2014).
[45] *Bitch Planet,* #3 (2015).
[46] Coates (2015).
[47] Freedman & Combs (1996).
[48] Goodman & Kivel (2020, June 12); McIntosh (1989).
[49] Crenshaw (2019).
[50] Crenshaw, et al. (1996).
[51] Maggs (2015).
[52] Campbell (2019, June 19).
[53] Holland (2018, June 7).
[54] Holland (2018, June 7).
[55] Crenshaw, et al. (1996).
[56] Maurer, et al. (2017, March 19).
[57] Blow (2008).
[58] Dontnod Entertainment (2015).
[59] Minority Media (2012).
[60] Sugar, et al. (2013–2019).
[61] *Ghost in the Shell,* vol. 1 (1989/2004).
[62] Lorde (2017), p. 228.
[63] Adorno et al. (2007).

[64] Miserandino (2003).
[65] Kershner (1980).
[66] CD Projekt Red (2015).
[67] Singleton (2010).

Chapter 3

[68] Goodhartz et al. (1991).
[69] Dante (1984).
[70] White (2007).
[71] Nickerson (1998).
[72] McKay, et al. (2007); Linehan (2015).
[73] American Psychiatric Association (2013).
[74] *Akira,* vol. 1, #1 (1988).
[75] Otomo (1988).
[76] Matt Makes Games (2018).
[77] *X-Men,* vol. 1, #101 (1976).
[78] American Psychiatric Association (2013).
[79] Rowling (1999b).
[80] Duffer, et al. (2016–current).
[81] White (2007).
[82] Bithell (2012).
[83] Zaslove (1988, January 24).
[84] Infinite Fall (2017).
[85] Miyazaki (2001).
[86] Whedon (2012).
[87] Rowling (1999a).
[88] Dante (1990).

Chapter 4

[89] Gamble, et al. (2016, January 25).
[90] Tolkien (1954/1994a).
[91] Kilmer, et al. (2014).
[92] Tedeschi, et al. (2018).
[93] Klasen, et al. (2010); Garski & Mastin (2019b)
[94] Arad, et al. (1992–1997).
[95] *X-Man,* vol. 1, #1 (1995); *Weapon X* #1 (1995).
[96] *X-Factor*, vol. 1, #68 (1991).

[97] Boothby, et al. (2006); Klasen et al. (2010).
[98] Smokowski, et al. (2000).
[99] Klasen, et al. (2010).
[100] Favreau, et al. (2019–present).
[101] Levine & Heller (2011); van der Kolk (2014/2015).
[102] Krull & Hewitt (1994).
[103] Rogers & Taff, (1968–2001).
[104] Roddenberry, et al. (1987–1994).
[105] Gardner & Knowles (2008).
[106] Madigan (2019); Bean (2019).
[107] *X-Men*, vol. 1, #102 (1976).
[108] *X-Men*, vol. 1, #117 (1979).
[109] *X-Men*, vol. 1, #102 (1976).
[110] Calhoun & Tedeschi (2006); Tedeschi et al. (2018).
[111] Van Slyke (2013).
[112] American Psychiatric Association (2013).
[113] Levine & Heller (2011).
[114] Boyd-Franklin (2003/2006).
[115] Benioff, et al. (2011–2019).
[116] Whedon, et al. (1997–2003).
[117] CD Projekt (2015).
[118] Bean (2018); Bean (2019).
[119] Frankl (1946/2006).
[120] CD Projekt (2015).
[121] Nintendo (1998).
[122] Nintendo (2000).
[123] Garski & Mastin (2019a)
[124] Thatgamecompany & Santa Monica Studio (2012).
[125] Campbell (1949/2008).
[126] *Uncanny X-Men*, vol. 1, #170 (1983).
[127] *Uncanny X-Men*, vol. 1, #325 (1995).
[128] Kornfield (2008).

Chapter 5

[129] Nolan, et al. (2018, June 24).
[130] Pierpont (1997, February 9).
[131] Duffield (1995–1997).
[132] Campbell (1959/1976).
[133] Alcaro & Carta (2019).

[134] Coppa (2017).
[135] Hellekson & Busse (2006).
[136] Jamison (2013).
[137] Jamison (2013).
[138] Rice (1974).
[139] White (2007).
[140] Nintendo (1998).
[141] Whedon (2000, May 23).
[142] Skir, et al. (1993, January 30).
[143] Krull & Hewitt (1994).
[144] Jamison (2013).
[145] Frankl (1946/2006).
[146] Spiegelman (1981–1990/1991).
[147] Frost & Lynch (1990–1991).
[148] Campbell (1964/1976).
[149] Coogler, 2018.

Chapter 6

[150] Reed, et al. (2016, March 7).
[151] Lord & Miller (2014).
[152] Gazso & McDaniel (2015).
[153] Rosaen & Dibble (2015).
[154] Stever (2017).
[155] Johnson (2017).
[156] Bridges (2006).
[157] *Wolverine*, vol. 3, #66 (2008).
[158] Clarkson, et al. (2015–2018).
[159] *Alias*, vol. 1, #4 (2002).
[160] Reed, et al. (2016, March 7).
[161] Brontë (1847/2002).
[162] Bioware (2010).
[163] Bioware (2012).

Chapter 7

[164] Jemison (2017), p. 166.
[165] Cahill, et al. (2015–2020).
[166] Satir (1990).

[167] Favreau, et al. (2019–present).
[168] Bowen (1985/2004).
[169] Minuchin & Fishman (1981).
[170] Macfie, et al. (2015).
[171] Whitaker, C. (1982); Whitaker C. A. (1989).
[172] Minuchin & Fishman (1981).
[173] Macfie, et al. (2015).
[174] Silver, et al. (2004–2007).
[175] Berman, et al. (1993–1999).
[176] Sherman-Palladino, et al. (2000–2007).
[177] Brooks, et al. (1992–present).
[178] Minuchin & Fishman (1981).
[179] Roddenberry, et al. (1987–1994).
[180] Minuchin & Fishman (1981).
[181] ConcernedApe (2016).
[182] Miyazaki (2001).
[183] Gatiss, et al. (2010–2017).
[184] Fuller et al. (2017–present).
[185] Chapman (1992/2015).
[186] Chapman (1992/2015).

Chapter 8

[187] Kripke (2008, May 15).
[188] Satir (1990).
[189] *The Wicked + The Divine*, #14 (2015); *The Wicked + The Divine: 1831* (2016).
[190] van der Kolk (2014/2015); Wolynn (2016).
[191] Weinhold (2006); Wolynn (2016).
[192] Salberg (2015).
[193] van der Kolk (2014/2015).
[194] Wolynn (2016).
[195] Menakem (2017).
[196] Menakem (2017); Wolynn (2016).
[197] Garski & Mastin (2019a).
[198] *Jungle Action*, #7 (1973).
[199] Coogler (2018).
[200] Boyd-Franklin (2003/2006).
[201] Spiegelman (1981–1990/1991).
[202] Morrison (1987).
[203] Menakem (2017).

[204] Tedeschi, et al. (2018).
[205] McGoldrick, et al. (1999).
[206] McGoldrick, et al. (1999).
[207] Bowen (1985/ 2004).
[208] Skowron (2004).
[209] Johnson (2019).
[210] Minuchin & Fishman (1981).
[211] Jung (1990b).
[212] Shankar (2015–present).
[213] Corey (2015).
[214] Corey (2015).
[215] Corey (2015).
[216] Shankar, et al. (2015–present).
[217] Corey (2011).
[218] Clarkson, et al. (2015–2018).
[219] Infinite Fall (2017).
[220] Braithwaite, et al. (2010); Voorpostel (2013).
[221] Harris, et al. (1985–1992).
[222] Hirsch (1994–1996).
[223] Miyazaki (1997).
[224] Krieger, et al. (2018–2020).
[225] *Chilling Adventures of Sabrina*, vol. 1 (2016).
[226] Pullman (1996).

Chapter 9

[227] Day & Evey (2007–2012).
[228] Madigan (2019), pp. 227–239; Bean (2018).
[229] Hull (2019).
[230] Stone (2019).
[231] Madigan (2019); Stone (2019).
[232] Campbell (2019, June 19).
[233] Campbell (2019, June 19).
[234] Prochaska & DiClemente (1984).
[235] Matz & Frankel (2004/2014).

Chapter 10

[236] Ames, et al. (2009, September 20).
[237] Tolkien (1954/1994b).

[238] *X-Men*, vol. 1, #65 (1970).
[239] *X-Men*, vol. 1, #65 (1970) & Skir, et al. (1994, January 8).
[240] *X-Men*, vol. 1, #94 (1975).
[241] Tolkien (1937/1994).
[242] Boden (2019).
[243] Jung (1990a).
[244] American Psychiatric Association (2013).
[245] Hays & Iwamasa (2006).
[246] Linehan (1993).
[247] Favreau (2010).
[248] Shapiro & Forrest (1997/2016).
[249] Nolan (2010).
[250] Schwartz (2001).
[251] White & Epston (1990/2015).
[252] McWilliams (2004).
[253] Satir (1990).

Chapter 11

[254] Jackson (2001).
[255] Linehan (2015).
[256] Collins (2008).
[257] Roth (2011).
[258] Jemison (2017).
[259] Butler (1991/2000).
[260] Mobius Digital (2019).
[261] Locke (1689/2016).
[262] Hobbes (1651/2017).
[263] Kübler-Ross & Kessler (2014).
[264] Kübler-Ross (1969).
[265] Whedon (2001, February 27).
[266] Kübler-Ross (1969).
[267] Kessler (2019).
[268] The Intergovernmental Panel on Climate Change (2018, October 8).
[269] Heyward (1990–1996).
[270] Mosenberg (2018, July 24).
[271] Schwartz, et al. (2006, November 2).
[272] L'Engle (1962; 1973; 1978).
[273] Jackson (2001).
[274] Schur (2020, January 30).

[275] Horkheimer & Adorno (1947/2002).

[276] Braga, et al. (1994, May 23).

Chapter 12

[277] Gewirtz, et al. (2010, May 13).

[278] Rowling (1998), p. 50.

[279] Rowling (1999a), p. 264.

[280] Braga, et al. (1994, May 23).

[281] Frost & Lynch (1990–1991).

[282] Rowling (1999b).

[283] Waititi (2017).

[284] Campbell (1959/1976); Campbell (1968/1976).

[285] van der Kolk (2014/2015).

[286] Leterrier, et al. (2019–present).

[287] Henson (1982).

References

Abrams, J. J., Nolan, J., Joy, L., Weintraub, J., Burk, B., Lewis, R. J., Patino, R., Wickham, A., Stephenson, B., & Thé, D. (Executive Producers). (2016–present). *Westworld* [TV series]. HBO Entertainment; Kilter Films; Bad Robot Productions; Jerry Weintraub Productions; Warner Bros. Television.

Adorno, T., Benjamin, W., Block, E., Brecht, B., & Lukács, G. (2007). *Aesthetics and Politics.* Verso.

Akinyela, M. (2002) De-colonizing our lives: Divining a post-colonial therapy. *The International Journal of Narrative Therapy and Community Work, 2002*(2), 32–43.

Akira, vol. 1, #1 (1988). "Chapter 1: The highway." Script: K. Otomo. Art: K. Otomo.

Alcaro, A., & Carta, S. (2019). The "instinct" of imagination. A neuro-ethological approach to the evolution of the reflective mind and its application to psychotherapy. *Frontiers in Human Neuroscience, 12*(522), 1–20. https://doi.org/10.3389/fnhum.2018.00522.

Alias, vol. 1, #4 (2002). Script: B. M. Bendis. Art: M. Gaydso.

Alias, vol. 1, #6 (2002). Script: B. M. Bendis. Art: M. Gaydso.

American Psychiatric Association. (2013). *Diagnostic and Statistical Manual of Mental Disorders* (5th ed.). American Psychiatric Association.

Ames, J. (Writer). Taylor, A. (Director). (2009, September 20). Stockholm syndrome. (Season 1, Episode 1) [TV series episode]. In J. Ames, S. Condon, S. Davis, D. Becky, & T. Miller (Executive Producers), *Bored to Death.* Dakota Pictures; 3 Arts Entertainment; Fair Harbor Productions; HBO Entertainment.

Arad, A., Lee, S., Calamari, J., Richard, W., & Rollman, E. S. (Executive Producers). (1992–1997). *X-Men: The Animated Series.* [TV series]. Marvel Entertainment Group; Saban Entertainment; Graz Entertainment; AKOM.

Bacon, L., & Aphramor, L. (2011). Weight science: Evaluating the evidence for a paradigm shift. *Nutrition Journal, 10*(9). https://doi.org/10.1186/1475-2891-10-9.

Bacon-Smith, C. (1992). *Enterprising Women: Television Fandom and the Creation of Popular Myth*. University of Pennsylvania Press.

Bean, A. M. (2018). *Working with Video Gamers and Games in Therapy: A Clinician's Guide*. Taylor & Francis Group.

Bean, A. M. (2019). I am my avatar and my avatar is me: Utilizing video games as therapeutic tools. In J. Stone (Ed.), *Integrating Technology into Modern Therapies: A Clinician's Guide to Developments and Interventions*. (1st ed.) (pp. 24–36). Taylor & Francis Group.

Benioff, D., Weiss, D. B., Strauss, C., Doelger, F., Caulfield, B., O'Roarke, I., Sapochnik, M., & Nutter, D. (Executive Producers). (2011–2019). *Game of Thrones* [TV series]. HBO Entertainment; Television 360; Grok! Television; Generator Entertainment; Startling Television; Bighead Littlehead.

Berger, P., & Luckmann, T. (1966). *The Social Construction of Reality: A Treatise in the Sociology of Knowledge*. Double Day.

Berman, R., Piller, M., & Behr, I. S. (Executive Producers). (1993–1999). *Star Trek: Deep Space Nine (DS9)* [TV series]. Paramount Domestic Television.

Bioware. (2007). *Mass Effect*. Microsoft Game Studios.

Bioware. (2010). *Mass Effect 2*. Electronic Arts.

Bioware. (2012). *Mass Effect 3*. Electronic Arts.

Bitch Planet #1 (2014). Script: K. S. DeConnick. Art: V. De Landro.

Bitch Planet #3 (2015). "Too Big to Fail." Script: K. S. DeConnick. Art: R. Wilson IV.

Bithell, M. (2012). *Thomas Was Alone*. Mike Bithell; Curve Digital; Bossa Studios.

Blow, J. (2008). *Braid*. Number None; Microsoft Game Studios.

Boden, A. (Director). (2019). *Captain Marvel* [Film]. Marvel Studios.

Boothby, N., Crawford, J., & Halperin, J. (2006). Mozambique child soldier life outcome study: Lessons learned in rehabilitation and reintegration efforts. *Global Public Health, 1*(1), 87–107. Doi: 10.1080/17441690500324347.

Bowen, M. (1985/2004). *Family Therapy in Clinical Practice*. Rowman & Littlefield Publishers.

Boyd-Franklin, N. (2003/2006). *Black Families in Therapy* (2nd ed., & Paperback ed.). Guilford Press.

Braga, B., (Writer), Moore, R. D. (Writer), & Kolbe, W. (Director). (1994, May 23). All good things . . . (Season 7, Episodes 25 & 26) [TV series episode]. In G. Roddenberry, R. Berman, M. Piller, & J. Taylor (Executive Producers), *Star Trek: The Next Generation*. Paramount Domestic Television.

Braithwaite, D. O., Wackernagel, B. B, Baxter, L. A., DiVerniero, R., Hammonds, J. R., Hosek, A. M., Willer, E. K., & Wolf, B. M. (2010). Constructing family: A typology of voluntary kin. *Papers in Communication Studies, 87*, 388–407. http://digitalcommons.unl.edu/commstudiespapers/87.

Bridges, M. R. (2006). Activating the corrective emotional experience. *Journal of Clinical Psychology: In Session, 62*(5), 551–568.

Briggs, K. C., & Myers, I. B. (1977). *Myers-Briggs Type Indicator: Form G Booklet.* Consulting Psychologists Press.

Brontë, E. (1847/2002). *Wuthering Heights.* (R. J. Dunn, Ed.) (4th ed.). W. W. Norton & Company.

Brooks, J. L., Groening, M., et al. (Executive Producers). (1992–present). *The Simpsons* [TV series]. Gracie Films; 20th Century Fox Television.

Buffy the Vampire Slayer Season Eight (2007–2011). Creator: J. Whedon. Art: G. Jeanty, K. Moline, & A. Owens.

Butler, O. E. (1991/2000). *Parable of the Sower.* Open Road Integrated Media.

Cahill, M., London, M., Williams, J., Smith, S., McNamara, J., Gamble, S., Reed, D., Fisher, C., Lieser, L., & Myers, H. A. (Executive Producers). (2015–2020). *The Magicians* [TV series]. McNamara Moving Company; Man Sewing Dinosaur; Groundswell Productions; Universal Cable Productions; Universal Content Productions.

Calhoun, L. G., & Tedeschi, R. G. (2006). The foundations of posttraumatic growth: An expanded framework. In L. G. Calhoun & R. G. Tedeschi (Eds.), *Handbook of Posttraumatic Growth: Research and Practice* (pp. 3–23). Lawrence Erlbaum Associates, Publishers.

Campbell, C. (2019, June 19). The Anita Sarkeesian story. *Polygon.* https://www.polygon.com/features/2019/6/19/18679678/anita-sarkeesian-feminist-frequency-interview-history-story.

Campbell, J. (1949/2008). *The Hero with a Thousand Faces* (3rd ed.). New World Library.

Campbell, J. (1959/1976). *The Masks of God: Primitive Mythology.* Penguin Books.

Campbell, J. (1962/1976). *The Masks of God: Oriental Mythology.* Penguin Books.

Campbell, J. (1964/1976). *The Masks of God: Occidental Mythology.* Penguin Books.

Campbell, J. (1968/1976). *The Masks of God: Creative Mythology.* Penguin Books.

CD Projekt Red. (2015). *The Witcher 3: Wild Hunt.* CD Projekt Red.

Chapman, G. (1992/2015). *The 5 Love Languages: The Secret to Love That Lasts.* Northfield Publishing.

Chilling Adventures of Sabrina, vol. 1 (2016). "The Crucible." Script: R. Aguirre-Sacasa. Art: R. Hack & J. Morelli.

Clarkson, S. J., Friedman, L., Goss, A., Henigman, K., Holland, C., Fine, A., Lee, S., Quesada, J., Buckley, D., Chory, J., Loeb, J., Rosenberg, M., Zreik, K., Bendis, B. M., Kenny, J., Klein, H., Reynolds, S., Hilly, H., & Tucker, R. (Executive Producers). (2015–2018). *Marvel's Jessica Jones* [TV series]. Marvel Television; ABC Studios; Tall Girls Productions.

Coates, Ta-Nehisi (2015). *Between the World and Me.* Spiegel & Grau.

Cohen, E. L. (2010). Expectancy Violations in Relationships with Friends and Media Figures. *Communication Research Reports, 27*(2), 97–111.

Cole, T., & Leets, L. (1999). Attachment styles and intimate television viewing: Insecurely forming relationships in a parasocial way. *Journal of Social and Personal Relationships, 16*(4), 495–511.

Collins, S. (2008). *The Hunger Games*. Scholastic Press.

ConcernedApe. (2016). *Stardew Valley* (Nintendo Switch). ConcernedApe; Chucklefish.

Coogler, R. (Director). (2018). *Black Panther* [Film]. Marvel Studios.

Coppa, F. (2017). *The Fanfiction Reader: Folktales for a Digital Age*. University of Michigan Press.

Corey, J. S. (2011). *Leviathan Wakes*. Orbit Books.

Corey, J. S. (2015). *Nemesis Games*. Orbit Books.

Crenshaw, K., Gotanda, N., Pellar, G., & Thomas, K. (Eds.). (1996). *Critical Race Theory: The Key Writings That Formed the Movement* (1st ed.) The New Press.

Crenshaw, K., Harris L. C., Hosang, D. M., & Lipsitz, G. (Eds.). (2019). *Seeing Race Again: Countering Colorblindness across the Disciplines* (1st ed.) University of California Press.

Dante, J. (Director). (1984). *Gremlins* [Film]. Warner Bros.; Amblin Entertainment.

Dante, J. (Director). (1990). *Gremlins 2: The New Batch* [Film]. Amblin Entertainment.

Day, F., & Evey, K. (Executive Producers). (2007–2012). *The Guild.* [Web series].

Dolynski, M. (Writer), & Alexander, D. (Director). (1968, November 22). Plato's Stepchildren. (Season 3, Episode 10) [TV series episode]. In G. Roddenberry (Executive Producer), *Star Trek: Original Series*. Desilu Productions; Norway Corporation; Paramount Television.

Dontnod Entertainment. (2015). *Life Is Strange (Steam).* Square Enix.

Duffer, M. Duffer, R. Levy, S. Cohen, D., Holland, C. Wright, B., Thunell, M, Gaidusek, K., Gwin, C., & Paterson, I. (Executive Producers). (2016–2021). *Stranger Things* [TV series]. 21 Laps Entertainment; Monkey Massacre.

Duffield, R. (Executive Producer). (1995–1997). *Wishbone* [TV series]. Big Feats! Entertainment.

Eyal, K., & Dailey, R. M. (2012). Examining relational maintenance in parasocial relationships. *Mass Communication and Society, 15*(5), 758–781.

Fanon, F. (2005). *The Wretched of the Earth* (R. Philcox, Trans.). Grove Press. (Original work published 1963).

Fanon, F. (2008). *Black Skin, White Masks* (R. Philcox, Trans.). Grove Press. (Original work published 1967).

Favreau, J. (Director). (2010). *Iron Man 2* [Film]. Marvel Studios.

Favreau, J., Filoni, D., Kennedy, K., & Wilson, C. (Executive Producers). (2019–present). *The Mandalorian* [TV series]. Lucasfilm; Fairview Entertainment; Golem Creations.

Frankl, V. (1946/2006). *Man's Search for Meaning*. Beacon Press.

Freedman, J., & Combs, G. (1996). *Narrative Therapy: The Social Construction of Preferred Realities*. W. W. Norton & Co.

Frost, D., & Lynch, D. (Executive Producers). (1990–1991). *Twin Peaks* [TV series]. Lynch/Frost Productions; Propaganda Films; Spelling Television; Twin Peaks Productions.

Fuller, B., Semel, D., Roddenberry, R., Roth, T., Goldsmann, A., Kadin, H., Berg, G., Harberts, A., Willmott, V., Duff, J., Osunsanmi, O., Weber, J., Siracusa, F., & Kurtzman, A. (Executive Producers). (2017–present). *Star Trek: Discovery* [TV series]. Secret Hideout; Roddenberry Entertainment; Living Dead Guy Productions; CBS Television Studios.

Gamble, S., McG, Kripke, E., Singer, R., et al. (Executive Producers). (2005–2020). *Supernatural* [TV series]. Kripke Enterprises; Wonderland Sound and Vision; Warner Bros. Television Distribution.

Gamble, S. (Writer), & Smith, S. (Director). (2016, January 25). The Source of Magic (Season 1, Episode 2) [TV series]. In M. Cahill, M. London, J. Williams, S. Smith, J. McNamara, S. Gamble, D. Reed, C. Fisher, L. Lieser, & H.A. Myers (Executive Producers). *The Magicians*. McNamara Moving Company; Man Sewing Dinosaur; Groundswell Productions; Universal Cable Productions; Universal Content Productions.

Gardner, W. L., & Knowles, M. L. (2008). Love makes you real: Favorite television characters are perceived as "real" in a social facilitation paradigm. *Social Cognition*, *26*(2), 156–168.

Garski, L., & Mastin, J. (2019a) Divided by our fathers: Transgenerational trauma in Black Panther. In T. Langley & A. Simmons (Eds.) *Black Panther Psychology: Hidden Kingdoms* (pp. 181–190) Sterling.

Garski, L., & Mastin, J. (2019b). The protective power of destiny: Posttraumatic growth in the Legend of Zelda. In A. Bean (Ed.) *The Psychology of Zelda* (pp. 131–150). BenBella Books.

Garski, L., & Mastin, J. (2020). Beyond canon: Therapeutic fanfiction and the queer hero's journey. In L. C. Ruben (Ed.) *Using Superheroes and Villains in Counseling and Play Therapy* (pp. 264–273). Routledge.

Gatiss, M., Moffat, S., Vertue, B., Eaton, R., Jones, R., & Vertue, S. (Executive Producers). (2010–2017). *Sherlock* [TV series]. Hartswood Films; BBC Walves; WGBH.

Gazso, A., & McDaniel, S. A. (2015). Families by choice and the management of low income through social supports. *Journal of Family Issues*, *36*(3), 371–395. https://psycnet.apa.org/doi/10.1080/15205436.2011.616276.

Gewirtz, E., & Kripke, E. (Writers) & Boyum, S. (Director). (2010, May 13). Swan Song (Season 4, Episode 22). [TV series episode]. In S. Gamble, McG, E. Kripke, & R. Singer, et al. (Executive Producers). (2005–2020). *Supernatural*. Kripke Enterprises; Wonderland Sound and Vision; Warner Bros. Television Distribution.

Ghost in the Shell, vol. 1 (1989/2004). Script: S. Masamune. Art: S. Masamune.

Goodhartz, S., Douglas, P., & Jones, R. (Writers) & Landau, L. (Director). (1991, May 18). Night Terrors (Season 4, Episode 17) [Television series episode]. In G. Roddenberry, R. Berman, M. Piller, & J. Taylor (Executive Producers). *Star Trek: The Next Generation*. Paramount Domestic Television.

Goodman, D., & Kivel, P. (2020). Oppression and Privilege Self-Assessment Tool. California Partnership to End Domestic Violence, 2020. https://www.cpedv.org/sites/main/files/oppression_and_privilegeself_assessment.pdf.

Goodyear Brown, P., & Gott, E. (2019). Tech, trauma work, and the power of titration. In J. Stone (Ed.), *Integrating Technology into Modern Therapies: A Clinician's Guide to Developments and Interventions*. (1st ed.). (pp. 109–123). Taylor & Francis Group.

Harris, S., Witt, J. P., Satkin, M., & Thomas, T. (Executive Producers). (1985–1992). *The Golden Girls* [TV series]. Witt/Thomas/Harris Productions; Buena Vista Television.

Hays, P. A., & Iwamasa, G. Y. (2006). *Culturally Responsive Cognitive Behavioral Therapy: Assessment, Practice, and Supervision.* American Psychological Association.

Headington Institute (2020, July 9). Self-Care and Lifestyle Balance Inventory (Self-Test) [Survey]. https://www.headington-institute.org/resource/self-care-inventory/.

Hellekson, K., & Busse, K. (2006). *Fan Fiction and Fan Communities in the Age of the Internet*. McFarland & Company, Inc.

Henson, J. (Director). (1982). *Dark Crystal* [Film]. Henson Associates; ITC Entertainment.

Heyward, A., London, R., Pyle, B., Boxer, N., Devreemtoes, B., Selbert, F., Potamking, B., Hanng, W., Barbera, J., & Tuner, T. (Executive Producers). (1990–1996). *Captain Planet and the Planeteers* [TV series]. DIC Enterprises; Hanna-Barbera Cartoons.

Hirsch, M. (Executive Producer). (1994–1996). *Gargoyles* [TV series]. Walt Disney Television Animation; Jade Animation; Tama Productions.

Hobbes, T. (1651/2017). *Leviathan*. Penguin Classics.

Holland, L. (2018, June 7). Why are (some) Star Wars fans so toxic? *The Guardian*. https://www.theguardian.com/film/2018/jun/07/kelly-marie-tran-rose-why-are-some-star-wars-fans-so-toxic.

Horkheimer, M., & Adorno, T. W. (1947/2002). *Dialectic of Enlightenment*. (E. Jephcott, Trans.). (G.S. Noerr, Ed.). Stanford University Press.

Horton, D., & Wohl, R. R. (1956). Mass communication and para-social interaction. *Psychiatry, 19*(3), 215–299.

Hull, K. (2019). Replace hesitancy and doubt with competency and skill: The technologically minded therapist. In J. Stone (Ed.), *Integrating Technology into Modern Therapies: A Clinician's Guide to Developments and Interventions*. (1st ed.). (pp. 24–36). Taylor & Francis Group.

Infinite Fall. (2017). *Night in the Woods, Weird Autumn Edition*. Finji.

The Intergovernmental Panel on Climate Change. (2018, October 8). Summary for Policymakers of IPCC Special Report on Global Warming of 1.5°C approved by governments. https://www.ipcc.ch/2018/10/08/summary-for-policymakers-of-ipcc-special-report-on-global-warming-of-1-5c-approved-by-governments/.

Jackson, P. (Director). (2001). *The Lord of the Rings: The Fellowship of the Ring*. New Line Cinema; WingNut Films.

Jamison, A. (2013). *Fic: Why Fan Fiction is Taking Over the World*. Smart Pop.

Jemison, N. K. (2017). *The Broken Earth Book Three: The Stone Sky*. Orbit Book Group.

Jenkins, H. (1992/2013). *Textual Poachers* (20th anniversary ed.). Routledge.

Johnson, R. (Director). (2017). *Star Wars: The Last Jedi* [Film]. Lucasfilm Ltd.

Johnson, R. (Director). (2019). *Knives Out* [Film]. MRC; T-Street.

Jung, C. G. (1990a). *The Collected Works of C.G. Jung: The Archetypes and the Collective Unconscious*. (R. F. C. Hull, Trans.). (Sir H. Read, M. Fordham, G. Adler, & W. McGuire, Eds.). (2nd ed., Vol. 9, Part 1). Princeton University Press. (Original work published 1969).

Jung, C. G. (1990b). *The Collected Works of C.G. Jung: Aion: Researches into the Phenomenology of Self* (R. F. C. Hull, Trans.), (Sir H. Read, M. Fordham, G. Adler, & W. McGuire, Eds.), (2nd ed., Vol. 9, Part 2). Princeton University Press. (Original work published 1969).

Jung, C. G. (2009). *The Red Book, Liber Novus* (S. Shamdasani, Ed.), (M. Kyburz, J. Peck, & S. Shamdasani, Trans.). W. W. Norton & Company.

Jungle Action #7 (1973). "Death Regiments Beneath Wakanda." Script: D. McGregor. Art: R. Buckler & K. Janson.

Ker, J. (1993). *A Most Dangerous Method: The Story of Jung, Freud, and Sabina Spielrein*. Vintage.

Kershner, I. (Director). (1980). *Star Wars: Episode V, The Empire Strikes Back*. [Film]. Lucasfilm.

Kessler, D. (2019). *The Sixth Stage of Grief.* Scribner.

Kilmer R. P., Gil-Rivas V., Griese B., Hardy S. J., Hafstad G. S., & Alisic E. (2014). Posttraumatic growth in children and youth: Clinical implications of an emerging research literature. *American Journal of Orthopsychiatry, 84*(5), 506–518. http://dx.doi.org/10.1037/ort0000016.

Klasen, F., Daniels, J., Oettingen, G., Post, M., & Hoyer, C. (2010). Posttraumatic resilience in Ugandan child soldiers. *Child Development, 81*(4), 1096–1113.

Kornfield, J. (2008). *The Art of Forgiveness, Lovingkindness, and Peace.* Bantam Dell.

Krieger, L. T., Goldwater, J., Schechter, S., Aguirre-Sacasa, R., & Berlanti, G. (Executive Producers). (2018–2020). *Chilling Adventures of Sabrina* [TV series]. Archie Comics; Warner Bros. Television; Berlanti Productions; Muckle Man Productions.

Kripke, E. (Writer). Manners, K. (Director). (2008, May 15). No Rest for the Wicked (Season 3, Episode 16) [TV series episode]. In S. Gamble, McG, E. Kripke, & R. Singer, et al. (Executive Producers). (2005–2020). *Supernatural.* Kripke Enterprises; Wonderland Sound and Vision; Warner Bros. Television Distribution.

Krull, K., & Hewitt, K. (1994). *Lives of the Writers: Comedies, Tragedies, and What the Neighbors Thought.* Harcourt Brace & Company.

Kübler-Ross, E. (1969). *On Death and Dying.* Macmillan.

Kübler-Ross, E., & Kessler, D. (2014). *On Grief and Grieving: Finding the Meaning of Grief through the Five Stages of Loss.* (Kindle version). Retrieved from amazon.com.

L'Engle, M. (1962). *A Wrinkle in Time.* Bantam Doubleday Dell Books for Young Readers.

L'Engle, M. (1973). *A Wind in the Door.* Bantam Doubleday Dell Books for Young Readers.

L'Engle, M. (1978). *A Swiftly Tilting Planet.* Bantam Doubleday Dell Books for Young Readers.

Leterrier, L., Henson, L., & Stanford, H. (Executive Producers). (2019–present). *The Dark Crystal: Age of Resistance.* [TV series]. The Jim Henson Company.

Levine, A., & Heller, R. (2011). *Attached: The New Science of Adult Attachment and How It Can Help You Find—and Keep—Love.* Tarcher Perigee.

Linehan, M. M. (1993). *Cognitive-Behavioral Treatment for Borderline Personality Disorder.* The Guilford Press.

Linehan, M. M. (2015). *DBT Skills Training Handouts and Worksheets* (2nd ed.). The Guilford Press.

Locke, J. (1689/2016). *The First & Second Treatises of Government.* Pantianos Classics. (Original work published 1689).

Lord, P., & Miller, C. (2014). *The LEGO Movie* [Film]. Warner Animation Group; Lin Pictures; LEGO Group; Vertigo Entertainment; Village Roadshow Pictures.

Lorde, A. (1988/2017). *A Burst of Light and Other Essays*. Ixia Press.

Macfie, J., Brumariu, L. E., & Lyons-Ruth, K. (2015). Parent–child role-confusion: A critical review of an emerging concept. *Developmental Review 36*(2015), 34–57.

Madigan, J. (2019). *Getting Gamers: The Psychology of Video Games and Their Impact on the People Who Play Them*. Rowman & Littlefield.

Maggs, S. (2015). *The Fangirl's Guide to the Galaxy: A Handbook for Girl Geeks*. Quirk Books.

Matt Makes Games. (2018). *Celeste*. Matt Makes Games.

Matz, J., & Frankel, E. (2004/2014). *Beyond a Shadow of a Diet: The Therapist's Guide to Treating Compulsive Eating*. Routledge.

Maurer, J., Twiss, J., Weiner, J. (Writers) & Werner, C. (Director). (2017, March 19). Federal Budget (Season 4, Episode 6) [TV series episode]. In J. Oliver, T. Carvell, L. Stanton, J. Taylor, & J. Thoday (Executive Producers), *Last Week Tonight*. Avalon Television; Partially Important Productions.

McGoldrick, M., Gerson, R., & Shellenberger, S. (1999). *Genograms: Assessment and Intervention* (2nd ed.). Norton.

McIntosh, P. (1989). White Privilege: Unpacking the Invisible Knapsack. National Seed Project. https://www.nationalseedproject.org/Key-SEED-Texts/white-privilege-unpacking-the-invisible-knapsack.

McKay, M., Wood, J., & Brantley, J. (2007). *The Dialectical Behavior Therapy Skills Workbook: Practical DBT Exercises for Learning Mindfulness, Interpersonal Effectiveness, Emotion Regulation, and Distress Tolerance*. New Harbinger Publications.

McWilliams, N. (2004). *Psychoanalytic Psychotherapy: A Practitioner's Guide*. The Guilford Press.

Menakem, R. (2017). *My Grandmother's Hands: Racialized Trauma and the Pathway to Mending Our Hearts and Bodies*. Central Recovery Press.

Minority Media. (2012). *Papo & Yo*. Minority Media.

Minuchin, S., & Fishman, H. C. (1981). *Family Therapy Techniques*. Harvard University Press.

Miserandino, C. (2003). The spoon theory. But you don't look sick: Stories behind the smiles. *But You Don't Look Sick*. https://butyoudontlooksick.com/articles/written-by-christine/the-spoon-theory/.

Miyazaki, H. (1997). *Princess Mononoke*. [Film]. Studio Ghibli.

Miyazaki, H. (2001). *Spirited Away*. [Film]. Studio Ghibli.

Mobius Digital (2019). *Outer Wilds*. Annapurna Interactive.

Morrison, T. (1987). *Beloved*. Alfred A. Knopf.

Mosenberg, D. (2018, July 24). The dirty truth is your recycling may actually end up in landfills. *MotherJones*. https://www.motherjones.com/politics/2018/07/the-dirty-truth-is-your-recycling-may-actually-go-to-landfills/.

Napier, A. Y., & Whitaker, C. (1978/2017). *The Family Crucible: The Intense Experience of Family Therapy*. Harper & Row.

Nickerson, R. (1998). Confirmation bias: A ubiquitous phenomenon in many guises. *Review of General Psychology, 2*(2), 175–220.

Nintendo. (1992). *The Legend of Zelda: A Link to the Past*. Nintendo.

Nintendo. (1998). *The Legend of Zelda: Ocarina of Time*. Nintendo.

Nintendo. (2000). *The Legend of Zelda: Majora's Mask*. Nintendo.

Nintendo. (2016). *The Legend of Zelda: Breath of the Wild*. Nintendo.

Nolan, C. (Director). (2010). *Inception* [Film]. Legendary Pictures; Syncopy.

Nolan, J., Joy, L. (Writers) & Toye, F. E. O. (Director). (2018, June 24). The Passenger (Season 2, Episode 10) [TV series episode]. In J. J. Abrams, J. Nolan, L. Joy, J. Weintraub, B. Burk, R. J. Lewis, R. Patino, A. Wickham, B. Stephenson & D. Thé. (Executive Producers), *Westworld*. HBO Entertainment; Kilter Films; Bad Robot Productions; Jerry Weintraub Productions Warner Bros. Television.

Otomo, K. (Director). (1988). *Akira* [Film]. Tokyo Movie Shinsha.

Pierpont, C. R. (1997, February 9). A society of one: Zora Neale Hurston, American contrarian. *New Yorker*. https://www.newyorker.com/magazine/1997/02/17/a-society-of-one.

Pillar, M. (Writer) & Bole, K. (Director). (June 18, 1990). The Best of Both Worlds, Part 1 (Season 3, Episode 26) [TV series episode]. In G. Roddenberry, R. Berman, M. Piller & J. Taylor (Executive Producers) *Star Trek: The Next Generation*. Paramount Domestic Television.

Pillar, M. (Writer) & Bole, K. (Director). (September 24, 1990). The Best of Both Worlds, Part 2 (Season 4, Episode 1) [TV series episode]. In G. Roddenberry, R. Berman, M. Piller & J. Taylor (Executive Producers) *Star Trek: The Next Generation*. Paramount Domestic Television.

Pitts, M., Joy, L. (Writers) & Lewis, R. J. (Director). (March 22, 2020). The Winter Line (Season 3, Episode 2) [TV series episode]. In J. J. Abrams, J. Nolan, L. Joy, J. Weintraub, B. Burk, R. J. Lewis, R. Patino, A. Wickham, B. Stephenson & D. Thé. (Executive Producers), *Westworld*. HBO Entertainment; Kilter Films; Bad Robot Productions; Jerry Weintraub Productions Warner Bros. Television.

Prochaska, J. O., & DiClemente, C. C. (1984). *The Transtheoretical Approach: Towards a Systematic Eclectic Framework*. Dow Jones Irwin.

Pullman, P. (1996). *The Golden Compass*. Alfred A. Knopf.

Reed, D. (Writer). Eliasberg, J. (Director). (2016, March 7). The Strangled Heart (Season 1, Episode 8) [TV series episode]. In M. Cahill, M. London, J. Williams, S. Smith, J. McNamara, S. Gamble, D. Reed, C. Fisher, L. Lieser, & H. A. Myers (Executive Producers). *The Magicians*. McNamara Moving Company; Man Sewing Dinosaur; Groundswell Productions; Universal Cable Productions; Universal Content Productions.

Remedy Entertainment. (2019). *Control*. 505 Games.

Rice, A. (1974). *Interview with the Vampire*. Knopf.

Roddenberry, G. (Executive Producer). (1966–1969). *Star Trek: Original Series* [TV series]. Desilu Productions; Norway Corporation; Paramount Domestic Television.

Roddenberry, G., Berman, R., Piller, M., & Taylor, J. (Executive Producers). (1987–1994). *Star Trek: The Next Generation* [TV series]. Paramount Domestic Television.

Rogers, F., & Taff, P. K. (Executive Producers). (1968–2001). *Mister Rogers' Neighborhood* [TV series]. WQED; Small World Enterprises; Family Communications, Inc.

Rosaen, S. F., & Dibble, J. L. (2015). Clarifying the role of attachment and social compensation on parasocial relationships with television characters. *Communication Studies, 67*(2), 147–162.

Roth, V. (2011). *Divergent*. Katherine Tegen Books.

Rothfuss, P. (2007). *The Name of the Wind: The Kingkiller Chronicle Day One*. Daw Books.

Rothfuss, P. (2011). *The Wise Man's Fear: The Kingkiller Chronicle Day Two*. Daw Books.

Rowling, J. K. (1998). *Harry Potter and the Sorcerer's Stone*. Bloomsberry.

Rowling, J. K. (1999a). *Harry Potter and the Chamber of Secrets*. Scholastic.

Rowling, J. K. (1999b). *Harry Potter and the Prisoner of Azkaban*. Scholastic.

Salberg, J. (2015). The texture of traumatic attachment: Presence and ghostly absence in transgenerational transmission. *Psychoanalytic Quarterly, 84*(1), 21–46.

Satir, V. (1990). *The New Peoplemaking* (2nd ed.). Science & Behavior Books.

Schur, M. (Writer & Director). (2020, January 30). Whenever You're Ready (Season 4, Episodes 13 & 14). [TV series episode]. In M. Schur, D. Miner, M. Sackett, & D. Goddard. (Executive Producers), *The Good Place*. Fremulon; 3 Arts Entertainment; Universal Television.

Schwartz, J., Savage, S. (Writers), & Toynton, I. (Director). (2006, November 2). The Avengers (Season 4, Episode 1) [TV series episode]. In D. Bartis, B. DeLaurentis, D. Liman, McG, S. Savage, & J. Schwartz. (Executive Producers), *The O.C.* College Hill Pictures; Wonderland Sound and Vision; Hypnotic; Warner Bros. Television.

Schwartz, R. C. (2001). *Internal Family Systems Model.* Trailheads Publications.

Shapiro, F., & Forrest, M. S. (1997/2016). *EMDR: The Breakthrough Therapy for Overcoming Anxiety, Stress, and Trauma* (Updated ed.). Basic Books.

Shankar, N., Fergus, M., Otsby, H., Daniel, S., Brown, J. F., Hall, S., Johnson, B., Kosove, A., Lancaster, L., Abraham, D., Franck, T., McDonough, T., & Nowak, D. (Executive Producers). (2015–present). *The Expanse* [TV series]. Penguin in a Parka; SeanDanielCO; Alcon Entertainment; Just So; Hivemind; Amazon Studios.

Sherman-Palladino, A., Palladino, D., Polone, G., & Rosenthal, D. S. (Executive Producers). (2000–2007). *Gilmore Girls* [TV series]. Dorothy Parker Drank Here Productions; Hofflund/Polone; Warner Bros. Television.

Siega, M., Girolamo, G., Morgenstein, L., Schechter, S., Gamble, S., Berlanti, G., Krieger, L.T., Tree, S., & Foley, M. (Executive Producers). (2018–present). *You* [TV series]. Berlanti Productions; Alloy Entertainment; A&E Studios; Warner Horizon Television.

Silver, J., Etheridge, D., Thomas, R., Wright-Ruggiero, D., Gwartz, J., Stokdyk, D., & Bell, K. (Executive Producers). (2004–2007). *Veronica Mars* [TV series]. Stu Segall Productions; Silver Pictures Television; Rob Thomas Productions.

Singleton, M. (2010). *Yoga Body: The Origins of Modern Posture Practice.* Oxford University Press.

Skir, R. N., & Isenberg, M. (Writers). Houston, L. (Director). (1993, January 30). Captive Hearts (Season 1, Episode 5) [TV series episode]. In A. Arad, S. Lee, J. Calamari, W. Richard, & E. S. Rollman (Executive Producers), *X-Men: The Animated Series.* Marvel Entertainment Group; Saban Entertainment; Graz Entertainment; AKOM.

Skir, R. N., & Isenberg, M. (Writers). Houston, L., & Bowman, R. (Directors). (1994, January 8). A Rogue's Tale (Season 2, Episode 22) [TV series episode]. In A. Arad, S. Lee, J. Calamari, W. Richard, & E. S. Rollman (Executive Producers), *X-Men: The Animated Series.* Marvel Entertainment Group; Saban Entertainment; Graz Entertainment; AKOM.

Skowron, E. A. (2004). Differentiation of self, personal adjustment, problem solving, and ethnic group belonging among persons of color. *Journal of Counseling & Development, 82*(4), 447–456.

Smokowski, P. R., Reynolds, A. J., & Bezcruzko, N. (2000). Resilience and protective factors in adolescents: An autobiographical perspective from disadvantaged youth. *Journal of School Psychology, 37*(4), 425–448.

Spiegelman, A. (1981–1990/1991). *Maus.* Pantheon Books.

Stever, G. S. (2017). Evolutionary theory and reactions to mass media: Understanding parasocial attachment. *Psychology of Popular Media Culture, 6*(2), 95–102.

Stone, J. (Ed.). (2019). *Integrating Technology into Modern Therapies: A Clinician's Guide to Developments and Interventions* (1st ed.). Taylor & Francis Group.

Sugar, R., Moreland, W., Miller, B. A., Pelphrey, J., Sorcher, R., Lelash, C., & Wigzell, T. (Executive Producers). (2013–2019). *Steven Universe* [Television series]. Cartoon Network Studios.

Tedeschi, R. G., Shakespeare-Finch, J., Taku, K., & Calhoun, L. G. (2018). *Posttraumatic Growth: Theory, Research, and Application* (1st ed.). Routledge.

Thatgamecompany & Santa Monica Studio. (2012). *Journey*. Sony Computer Entertainment; Annapurna Interactive.

Tolkien, J. R. R. (1937/1994). *The Hobbit or There and Back Again*. (Revised ed.). Random House Publishing Group.

Tolkien, J. R. R. (1954/1994a). *The Lord of The Rings Part One: Fellowship of the Ring*. Random House Publishing Group.

Tolkien, J. R. R. (1954/1994b). *The Lord of The Rings Part Two: The Two Towers*. Random House Publishing Group.

Uncanny X-Men, vol. 1, #170 (1983). "Dancin' in the Dark." Script: C. Claremont. Art: P. Smith & B. Wiacek.

Uncanny X-Men, vol. 1, #325 (1995). "Generation of Evil." Script: S. Lobdell. Art: J. Madureira, T. Townsend, & M. Ryan.

van der Kolk, B. (2014/2015). *The Body Keeps the Score* (Reprint ed.). Penguin Books.

Van der Veer, R. (2011). Tatyana on the couch: The vicissitudes of psychoanalysis in Russia. In S. Salvatore & T. Zittoun (Eds.), *Cultural Psychology and Psychoanalysis: Pathways to Synthesis* (pp. 49–65). Information Age Publishing.

Van Slyke, J. (2013). Post-traumatic growth. *Naval Center for Combat and Operational Stress Control*. Retrieved from www.nccosc.navy.mil.

Voorpostel, M. (2013). Just like family: Fictive kin relationships in the Netherlands. *Journals of Gertontology, Series B: Psychological Sciences and Social Sciences, 68*(5), 816–824. https://doi.org/10.1093/geronb/gbt048.

Wachowski L., & Wachowski L. (Directors). (1999). *The Matrix* [Film]. Village Roadshow Pictures; Groucho II Film Partnership; Silver Pictures.

Waititi, T. (Director). (2017). *Thor: Ragnarok* [Film]. Marvel Studios.

Weapon X, vol. 1, #1 (1995). "Unforgiven Trespasses." Script: L. Hama. Art: A. Kubert, K. Kesel, D. Green, & C. Warner.

Weinhold B. (2006). Epigenetics: The science of change. *Environmental Health Perspectives, 114*(3), A160–7.

Whedon, J. (Writer & Director). (2000, May 23). Restless (Season 4, Episode 22) [TV series episode]. In J. Whedon, D. Greenwalt, M. Noxon, F. R. Kuzui, S. Gallin, G. Berman, & K. Kuzui (Executive Producers), *Buffy the Vampire*

Slayer. Mutant Enemy Productions; Sandollar Television; Kuzui Enterprise; 20th Century Fox Television.

Whedon, J. (Writer & Director). (2001, February 27). The Body (Season 5, Episode 16) [TV series episode]. In J. Whedon, D. Greenwalt, M. Noxon, F. R. Kuzui, S. Gallin, G. Berman, & K. Kuzui (Executive Producers), *Buffy the Vampire Slayer*. Mutant Enemy Productions; Sandollar Television; Kuzui Enterprise; 20th Century Fox Television.

Whedon, J. (2012). *The Avengers*. [Film]. Marvel Studios.

Whedon, J., Greenwalt, D., Noxon, M., Kuzui, F. R. , Gallin, S., Berman, G., & Kuzui, K. (Executive Producers). (1997–2003). *Buffy the Vampire Slayer* [Television Series]. Mutant Enemy Productions; Sandollar Television; Kuzui Enterprise; 20th Century Fox Television.

Whitaker, C. A. (1982). *From Psyche to System: The Evolving Therapy of Carl Whitaker.* (J. J. Neil, D.P. Kniskern, Eds.). The Guilford Family Therapy Press.

Whitaker C. A. (1989). *Midnight Musings of a Family Therapist.* (M. O. Ryan, Ed.). W. W. Norton.

Whitaker, C. A., & Bumberry, W. A. (1988). *Dancing with the Family: A Symbolic-Experiential Approach*. Brunner/Mazel Publishers.

White, M. (2007). *Maps of Narrative Practice*. W. W. Norton.

White, M., & Epston, D. (1990/2015). *Narrative Means to Therapeutic Ends*. W. W. Norton.

The Wicked + The Divine, #14 (2015). "The Re-Re-Remix." Script: K. Gillen. Art: J. McKelvie.

The Wicked + The Divine: 1831 (2016). "Modern Romance." Script: K. Gillen. Art: S. Hans.

Wolverine, vol. 3, #66 (2008). "Old Man Logan: Part 1." Script: M. Miller. Art: S. McNiven & D. Vines.

Wolynn, M. (2016). *It Didn't Start with You: How Inherited Family Trauma Shapes Who We Are and How to End the Cycle*. Penguin Random House.

X-Factor, vol. 1, #68 (1991). "Finale." Script: W. Portacio, J. Lee, & C. Claremont. Art: W. Portacio & A. Thibert.

X-Man, vol. 1, #1 (1995). "Breaking Away." Script: J. Loeb. Art: S. Skroce, M. Sellers, C. Smith, B. Larosa, & W. Conrad.

X-Men, vol. 1, #65 (1970). "Before I'd Be a Slave . . ." Script: D. O'Neil. Art: N. Adams & T. Palmer.

X-Men, vol. 1, #94 (1975). "The Doomsmith Scenario!" Script: C. Claremont & L. Wein. Art: D. Cockrum & B. McLeod.

X-Men, vol. 1, #101 (1976). "Like a Phoenix, From the Ashes." Script: C. Claremont. Art: D. Cockrum & F. Chiaramonte.

X-Men, vol. 1, #102 (1976). "Who Will Stop the Juggernaut?" Script: C. Claremont. Art: D. Cockrum & S. Grainger.

X-Men, vol. 1, #117 (1979). "Psi War." Script: C. Claremont & J. Byrne. Art: J. Byrne & T. Austin.

Zaslove, M., Ross, D., Magon, J., Talkington, B. (Writers), & Geurs, K. (Director). (1988, January 24). Friend, in Deed/Donkey for a Day (Season 1, Episode 2) [TV series episode]. In K. Geurs, K. Kessel, E. Ghertner, & R. Mooney (Producers), *The New Adventures of Winnie the Pooh*. Walt Disney Television Animation.

INDEX

ACKNOWLEDGMENTS

So many wonderful humans have helped us along the journey of writing this book. We would like to thank our fabulous editor, Shayna Keyles, the Gandalf to our Frodo and Sam: You saw a tweet and decided it had the makings of a book. Without you, we never could have made it this far. Thank you for your faith, inspiration, and insightful edits. This book couldn't have become what it is without you. To the entire team at North Atlantic Books who became the fellowship of *Starship Therapise,* thank you for your time, critiques, patience, and care. We were able to carry the ring because of each of you.

We would like to thank our illustrator, J, who brought our fever dreams to life and who patiently resketched Arya until she was just right. Way back at New York Comic Con–2018, we got the idea to ask you to be a part of this book (if we could get it off the ground). Thank you for saying yes to be our illustrator. We couldn't imagine this book without your art, wit, and whimsy.

Thank you to our teachers and mentors who got us started on this therapy journey: Anne Ramage, PsyD, LMFT, who brought Carl Whitaker, Sal Minuchin, Virginia Satir, Murray Bowen, and all the rest of the founders of marriage and family therapy to life; J. Philip Rosier Jr., PsyD, LMFT, who gave us each our first command; Patty Hlava, PhD, who believed in us even when we weren't sure if we believed in ourselves; Ginny D'Angelo, LMFT, LICSW, who taught us the power of the genogram; Travis Langley, PhD, who took us under his batwing and into the Psych Geek fold; Janina Scarlet, PhD, who inspires us to contribute to pop culture psychology every day; and last, but certainly not least, Lawrence Rubin, PhD, who championed our book when it was no more than a twinkle in our eyes. Thank you all for your encouragement, challenges, and humor. You each have helped us to be better therapists, writers, and humans.

A big thank you goes to our fabulous Beta(zoid) readers Ani Janzen, MPH, RDN, LD, Rose Nelson, Donyae Coles, Paige N. Reitz, LCSW, Britt Johnson, and Lisa Colburn. We appreciate your thoughtful comments, insightful questions, and patience. You made this book *more,* and we are genuinely grateful.

Where would we be without our Starfleet heroes who inspired us as children and helped us create the vast interfandom universe of the *Starship Therapise*? Thank you to Gene Roddenberry and all the cast, crew, and writers of *Star Trek: The Original Series* and *Star Trek: The Next Generation*. Your stories and characters continue to inspire us. Thank you especially to Marina Sirtis, known in the Star Trek universe as Counselor Deanna Troi. You taught an entire generation of children that feelings not only matter but also are the crucial component of our humanity. And you inspired us to become the therapists we are today.

All human families are complicated, and ours are no different. That being said, thank you to our parents who prized knowledge and education and passed these gifts onto us. To counter Tolstoy, all fur families are happy in their own unique way. Thank you to each of our fur family members, past, present, and future: Charlie, Bella, Taku, Kewa, Tarack, Chingachgook, Umitok, Anakpok, Cosette, Valjean, Uncas, Maximus, Lucilla, Gurdjieff, Hela, Thor, Meronym, Katsu, and Tali. You make life extraordinary. Finally, a big thank you goes to our respective romantic partners: Eli Mastin and Brian Edward Therens. To Eli for keeping us humble and reminding us once we got our book deal that "now you have to write it" and to Brian who engaged in numerous discussions over the years about the very topics now in this book, we love and appreciate you both so much.

We appreciate you, dear reader. May you live long and prosper.

ABOUT THE AUTHORS

Larisa A. Garski, LMFT, and Justine Mastin, LMFT, LADC, E-RYT 200, YACEP, met while they were in graduate school and have been co-conspirators ever since. They are research partners and co-chapter authors in numerous pop culture and psychology texts, including *Supernatural Psychology*, *Daredevil Psychology*, *Westworld Psychology*, *The Psychology of Zelda*, *Black Panther Psychology*, and *The Joker Psychology*. In addition, they contributed chapters to the academic text *Using Superheroes and Villains in Counseling and Play Therapy: A Guide for Mental Health Professionals*. Justine and Larisa cohost the podcast *Starship Therapise* and cowrite the *Psychology Today* blog of the same name. They have appeared at numerous pop culture conventions, teaching yoga and speaking on fan-wellness topics. Their work in the wellness field has been covered by such outlets as the *Wall Street Journal, SELF, Forbes,* Syfy, Geek and Sundry, USgamer, *Bustle,* and more. They can be reached at their website: www.starshiptherapise.com.

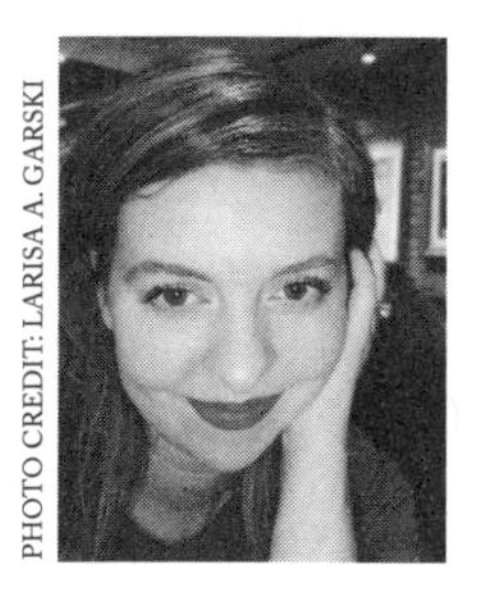

PHOTO CREDIT: LARISA A. GARSKI

Larisa A. Garski, MA, LMFT, is a psychotherapist and the clinical director at Empowered Therapy in Chicago, Illinois. She specializes in working with women, families, and young adults who identify as outside the mainstream, such as those in the geek and LGBTQIA+ communities.

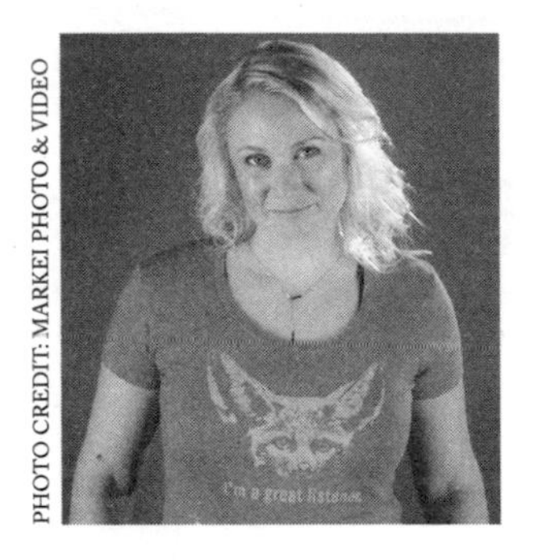
PHOTO CREDIT: MARKEI PHOTO & VIDEO

Justine Mastin, MA, LMFT, LADC, E-RYT 200, YACEP, is the owner and founder of Blue Box Counseling and is the creator and fearless leader of YogaQuest, a yoga organization that blends narratives with yoga and mindfulness. Justine also wrote the foreword to the self-published book *JSalvador's SuperEmoFriends: A Decade of Depression* and contributed an essay to the compilation *Embodied Resilience through Yoga: 30 Mindful Essays about Finding Empowerment after Addiction, Trauma, Grief, and Loss.* Justine is proud to take a holistic approach to healing: mind, body, and fandom.

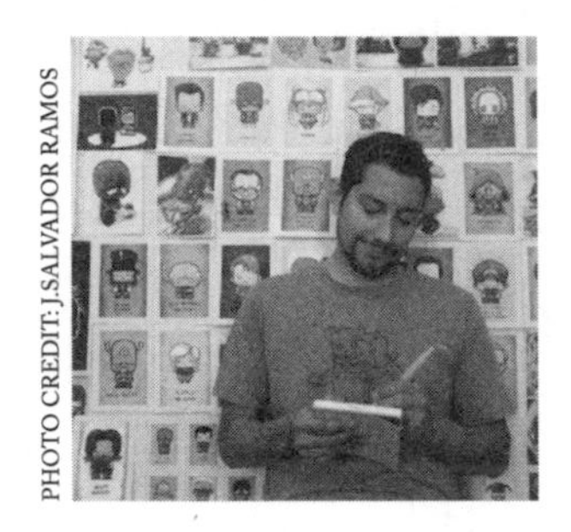
PHOTO CREDIT: J.SALVADOR RAMOS

J.Salvador Ramos is the cartoonist behind SuperEmoFriends, an ever-growing collection of satirical paintings inspired by the tragic events of popular culture. J. worked in motion graphics and animation in Hollywood, California, prior to the success of SuperEmoFriends.

About North Atlantic Books

North Atlantic Books (NAB) is an independent, nonprofit publisher committed to a bold exploration of the relationships between mind, body, spirit, and nature. Founded in 1974, NAB aims to nurture a holistic view of the arts, sciences, humanities, and healing. To make a donation or to learn more about our books, authors, events, and newsletter, please visit www.northatlanticbooks.com.

North Atlantic Books is the publishing arm of the Society for the Study of Native Arts and Sciences, a 501(c)(3) nonprofit educational organization that promotes cross-cultural perspectives linking scientific, social, and artistic fields. To learn how you can support us, please visit our website.